Home Care for the Client with Diabetes

Jetta Lee Fuzy, RN, MS
Director of Development and Training
Health Education, Incorporated
Fort Lauderdale, Florida

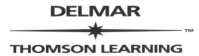

Africa • Australia • Canada • Denmark • Japan • Mexico • New Zealand • Philippines
Puerto Rico • Singapore • Spain • United Kingdom • United States

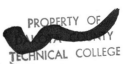

NOTICE TO THE READER

Cover Design by Brian J. Sullivan, Essinger Design Associates

Delmar Staff:

Publisher: Susan Simpfenderfer

Acquisitions Editor: Dawn Gerrain

Developmental Editor: Debra Flis

Project Editor: Elizabeth A. LaManna

Production Manager: Wendy A. Troeger

Team Assistant: Sandra Bruce

Art and Design Coordinator: Vincent S. Berger

Production Coordinator: John Mickelbank

Marketing Manager: Katherine Hans

Marketing Coordinator: Glenna Stanfield

Editorial Assistant: Donna L. Leto

COPYRIGHT © 1999 Delmar, a division of Thomson Learning, Inc. The Thomson Learning™ is a trademark used herein under license.

Printed in the United States of America
2 3 4 5 6 7 8 9 10 XXX 03 02 01 00

For more information, contact Delmar, 3 Columbia Circle, PO Box 15015, Albany, NY 12212-0515; or find us on the World Wide Web at http://www.delmar.com

International Division List

Asia
Thomson Learning
60 Albert Street, #15-01
Albert Complex
Singapore 189969
Tel: 65 336 6411
Fax: 65 336 7411

Japan:
Thomson Learning
Palaceside Building 5F
1-1-1 Hitotsubashi, Chiyoda-ku
Tokyo 100 0003 Japan
Tel: 813 5218 6544
Fax: 813 5218 6551

Australia/New Zealand:
Nelson/Thomson Learning
102 Dodds Street
South Melbourne, Victoria 3205
Australia
Tel: 61 39 685 4111
Fax: 61 39 685 4199

UK/Europe/Middle East
Thomson Learning
Berkshire House
168-173 High Holborn
London
WC1V 7AA United Kingdom
Tel: 44 171 497 1422
Fax: 44 171 497 1426

Latin America:
Thomson Learning
Seneca, 53
Colonia Polanco
11560 Mexico D.F. Mexico
Tel: 525-281-2906
Fax: 525-281-2656

Canada:
Nelson/Thomson Learning
1120 Birchmount Road
Scarborough, Ontario
Canada M1K 5G4
Tel: 416-752-9100
Fax: 416-752-8102

Spain:
Thomson Learning
Calle Magallanes, 25
28015-MADRID
ESPANA
Tel: 34 91 446 33 50
Fax: 34 91 445 62 18

Library of Congress Cataloging-in-Publication Data:

Fuzy, Jetta Lee.
    Home care for the client with diabetes / Jetta Lee Fuzy.
        p.   cm.
    Includes index.
    ISBN 0-8273-7935-8
    1. Diabetics—Home care. 2. Home health aides. I. Title.
    [DNLM: 1. Diabetes Mellitus. 2. Home Health Aides. 3. Home care
Services. WK 810 F996h 1998]
RC661.H63F89 1998
362.1'96462—dc21   98-18759
DNLM/DLC for Library of Congress   CIP

●Table of Contents

Preface v

Introduction vii

List of Procedures ix

Chapter 1   Anatomy and Physiology 1
Pancreas 2
Other Body Systems 3

Chapter 2   Overview of Diabetes 9
Types of Diabetes 10
Effects of Diabetes 12
Signs and Symptoms of Diabetes 13
Diagnosis of Diabetes 14

Chapter 3   Glucose Management and Control 17
Insulin Therapy 18
Oral Hypoglycemic Agents 21
Glucose Monitoring 23

Chapter 4   HCA Roles and Functions 27
Observation and Reporting 28
Documentation 31
HCA Care Plan 32
Home Care Aide Roles and Functions 34

Chapter 5   Acute Complications .39
Hypoglycemia 40
Ketoacidosis 41
Hyperglycemia 42
Insulin Shock 44

Chapter 6   Chronic Complications 47
Vascular Problems 48
Eye Disorders 49
Neuropathy 49
Infections 49
Skin Breakdown 50
Oral Hygiene 51
Stress 51
Other Illnesses 52

Chapter 7 Client Care 55
Foot Care 56
Skin Care 58
Bowel and Bladder Training 62
Collecting a Fresh, Fractional Urine Specimen 68
Testing Urine and Blood Sugar Levels 69
Disposal of Sharps 71

Chapter 8   Client and Family Education and Support 73
Disease Process 74
Diet 74
Complications 82
Exercise 83
Social Support 84

Chapter 9   Safety and Emergencies 87
Observing for Potential Risks 88
Maintaining a Safe Environment in the Home 90
Emergency Measures in Home Care 94
Infection Control 98

Chapter 10   Abuse 105
Six Types of Abuse 106
Reporting Abuse 107
Factors Contributing to Elderly Abuse 107
Signs of Elderly Abuse 108
Substance Abuse in the Elderly 110
Prevention 110

Chapter 11   Psychosocial Influences 113
The Holistic Model 114
Family Dynamics 116
Communication 117
Stresses on the Elderly Client 125
Behaviors of the HCA 126

Index 129

Preface

This specialty training module is designed to train the HCA to work with clients who have diabetes and who, for one reason or another, remain in the home. There are many aspects other than personal care involved in caring for clients with diabetes and their families. When the HCA is assigned to care for the client with diabetes in the home, the client has usually been newly diagnosed with diabetes, is unstable, or has undergone a recent change in medication. It is our intention in this program to educate the HCA with specific knowledge in the disease process in order for them to care for these special clients.

With less and less medical coverage available for long-term care for patients with diseases such as diabetes, the need for health care workers who have additional training will increase greatly in the next decade.

Chapter 1 contains a review of the anatomy and physiology of the nervous system that focuses on the endocrine system. An overview of diabetes is covered in Chapter 2. Chapter 3 discusses glucose management and control.

The roles and functions of the specially trained HCA, especially observation and reporting, is discussed in Chapter 4. Chapter 5 discusses acute complications of diabetes and Chapter 6 discusses its chronic complications. The procedures with which the HCA should be familiar when caring for a client with diabetes are discussed in Chapter 7 and include skin care, bowel and bladder training, foot care, collecting a fresh, fractional urine specimen, and blood glucose monitoring.

Education for clients and their families is the focus of Chapter 8. Safety and emergency situations, and their prevention, abuse issues, and psychosocial aspects of caring for these clients with diabetes are the focus of the last three chapters.

The HCA should also become an advocate for improving the care and medical coverage of this disease in the hopes of increasing funding for research, and eventually finding a cure for this serious and devastating illness.

ACKNOWLEDGMENTS

The author wishes to thank Jeleen Fuzy for her valuable input regarding both structure and content of this training manual. Without her patience and encouragement, I could not have completed this project.

The author and Delmar wish to thank the following individuals for reviewing the manuscript and providing valuable comments:

Rebecca Dierker-Bosco, RN, BSN
Director, Home Care Services
Tenet Home Care at Desert Hospital
Palm Springs, California

Kathy Kotlow, RN
Recruitment and Staff Development Manager
Olsten Kimberly Quality Care
Albany, New York

Kathy Lalley, RN
Clinical Manager
Yakima Valley Home Health
Toppenish, Washington

LaRae M. Ward, RN, MSN
OB/GYN Diabetes Educator
Dixie Regional Medical Center
Saint George, Utah

Introduction

Diabetes Mellitus is probably the most commonly seen disease in the home health care setting. It is estimated that over 14 million people are afflicted with Diabetes Mellitus, and more than half of these individuals do not realize they have it. These persons are two to six times more likely to have a heart attack or stroke, and more than half of them have high blood pressure. Diabetes is seen more often in Asian, Native, and African Americans than in Caucasians. And people who suffer from this disease are more likely to have the following health problems and complications:

- blindness
- foot and leg ulcers
- nerve-end damage in the hands and feet
- kidney problems
- infections
- poor healing ability
- poor circulation
- amputations (usually of the lower extremities)

Because there are many serious complications associated with diabetes, it is important for health care providers to educate the client and family in the disease process and return the client to self-care. It requires a team of home health professionals which include the physician, nurse, dietitian, and the HCA to care for and teach the diabetic client and family.

With the advent of Diagnostic Related Groups (DRGs) and early discharge from the hospital, home health nurses are more involved in early diabetes education, review, reinforcement of prior learning, supervision, and family and client support. The specially trained HCA may be expected to assist the nurse in this support process more and more in the future as clients are more frequently returned to their homes.

Newly diagnosed clients with diabetes may be discharged from the hospital before their diabetes education is complete. The home setting is much more conducive to learning, and the client and the family are more receptive to new information. The nurse begins the client education process by evaluating what the client and family already know. Education is vital to the stabilization of the diabetic client, and the physician and home health nurse are the primary educators, along with HCAs, who emphasize these teachings.

This training module focuses on the disease and the important aspects of care with which the HCA should be familiar in order to prepare to function properly in the specialty area of caring for the diabetic client at home. Most of the people seen in the home are either new diabetics or diabetics who are unstable, and need to be observed and monitored so that the symptoms can be managed and kept under control. The specially trained HCA should have a greater knowledge of this disease so that in situations requiring immediate action, intelligent choices can be made. In addition, greater knowledge will enable early preventative measures to be started, and life changes made to make a difference in the clients' well-being and future health.

Diabetes is a chronic disease, but clients can learn to live within its confines to lead normal lives. It is important for the HCA to help the client adjust to the change in lifestyle as quickly as possible, and lead as close to a normal life as possible.

The training module reviews the anatomy and physiology associated with diabetes. It is important to define this disease further in terms of types of diabetes, the signs and symptoms of each, the client care involved, acute and chronic complications, and most important, the home care aides' roles and functions. Finally, it discusses the importance of family and client education, support and community resources, and psychosocial influences.

List of Client Care Procedures

Procedure 1   Foot and Toenail Care
Procedure 2   Special Skin Care and Pressure Sores
Procedure 3   Training and Retraining Bowels
Procedure 4   Retaining the Bladder
Procedure 5   Collecting a Fresh, Fractional Urine Specimen
Procedure 6   Testing Urine for Acetone: Ketostix® Strip Test

Anatomy and Physiology

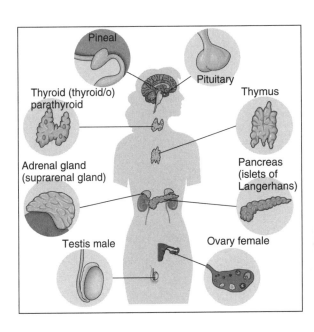

OBJECTIVES

Upon reading this chapter and completing the review questions, the home care aide (HCA) should be able to:

1. Define the endocrine system and its role in diabetes.

2. Describe the function of the pancreas and Islets of Langerhans.

3. Be familiar with how Diabetes Mellitus affects the nervous system, the cardiovascular system, and the urinary system.

KEY TERMS

glands	insulin
glucagon	Islets of Langerhans
hormones	

INTRODUCTION

The endocrine system is important to the specially trained HCA because it plays a major role in the physical and chemical process that keep the body in balance. When these chemical processes are out of balance, they can cause diseases such as diabetes. The endocrine system regulates chemical reactions that affect growth, reproduction, and metabolism (see Figure 1–1).

Figure 1–1 The Endocrine System

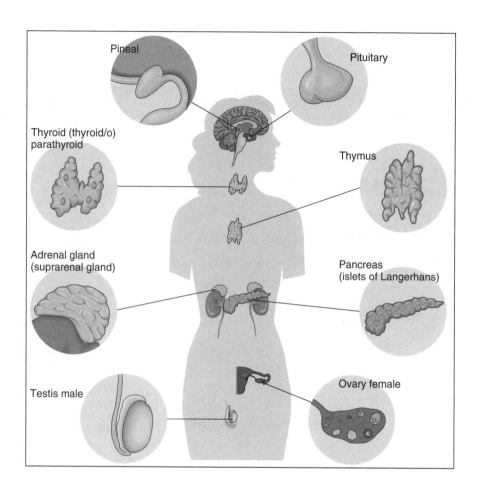

glands groups of cells that produce secretions.

hormones substances formed in glands and carried to organs or tissues to carry out specific bodily functions.

The endocrine system is a diverse system of **glands** and **hormones** (Figure 1–2). Endocrine glands are ductless glands that secrete chemical substances (hormones) directly into the bloodstream. These glands have a rich blood supply so that the hormones they produce can rapidly enter the bloodstream. The endocrine system includes the ovaries and testes, the pituitary gland, the thyroid gland, the parathyroid glands, the adrenal glands, and the pancreas. Table 1–1 shows the functions of each gland in the endocrine system.

PANCREAS

Islets of Langerhans cells in the pancreas which produce the hormones insulin and glucagon.

insulin hormone that helps the body utilize sugar and carbohydrates.

glucagon hormone that increases blood sugar and opposes the effects of insulin.

The pancreas lies behind the stomach, and is attached to the duodenum by ducts. The **Islets of Langerhans** are small groups of cells in the pancreas. There are approximately one million Islets of Langerhans in the pancreas scattered over the entire gland concentrated in the tail section. The Islets of Langerhans secrete **insulin** and **glucagon**.

In patients with diabetes, the pancreas does not produce enough insulin. Figure 1–3 shows how insulin enters the bloodstream. Because diabetes affects other systems of the body, the HCA should be familiar with a brief overview of them.

Table 1–1   Functions of the Glands of the Endocrine System

Pituitary gland	Secretes horomones which regulate many bodily processes; controlled by the hypothalamus.
Throid gland	Helps regulate the metabolic rate and growth process.
Parathyroid glands	Regulate metabolism of calcium and phosphorous.
Thymus gland	Regulates immunity to infectious disease during infancy and early childhood; becomes smaller as the body ages.
Adrenal glands	Adjust body to crisis and stress; increase blood pessure; speed reactions; metabolize carbohydrates and proteins.
Islets of Langerhans	Produce insulin necessary for the breakdown of glucose in the body.
Ovaries	Produce ovum (egg) for reproduction; secrete estrogen and progesterone which develop and maintain secondary sexual characteristics.
Testes	Produce sperm to fertilize ovum; secrete male hormone testosterone.

OTHER BODY SYSTEMS

The other body systems affected by diabetes are the nervous system, the cardiovascular system, and the urinary system. A brief overview of each of these and how diabetes affects each one is necessary in the education of the specially trained HCA.

The nervous system controls all activities of the body. It has two primary parts: the central nervous system, which includes the brain and the spinal cord; and the peripheral nervous system,

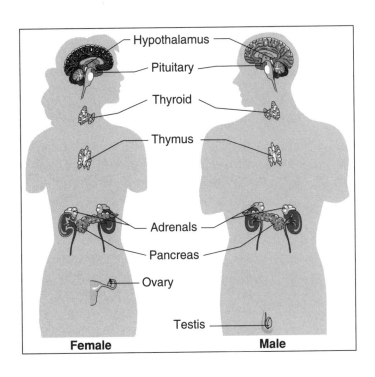

Figure 1–2 Structures of the Endocrine System

Figure 1–3 Insulin is a "bridge" that allows glucose to pass from the blood into body cells where it is used for energy. Insufficient insulin causes the glucose to remain in the blood.

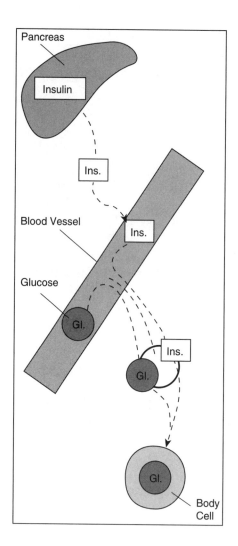

which includes the cranial and spinal nerves. Figure 1–4 shows the nervous system. The sensory organs are part of the nervous system and include the eyes, ears, nose, taste buds, and skin. In diabetics, the most common effects to the nervous system are damage to the retina of the eyes. Diabetes is the leading cause of new blindness in adults. In the peripheral nervous system, the client's legs are often affected. These clients present with symptoms which include loss of temperature sensation, pain, and numbness. Because of high glucose levels in the blood that are not under control, diabetic patients suffer from weakened leg muscles, making them more prone to injuries. In addition, cerebrovascular accidents (CVA), or strokes, are among the leading causes of death in clients with diabetes.

A disorder of the retina occurring in clients with diabetes is called diabetic retinopathy, and is caused by fragile blood vessels weakened by hypertension and high glucose levels. Fifty percent of juvenile diabetics develop this problem after ten to fifteen years. Treatment of neuropathy and retinal problems is to control the client's glucose levels.

Figure 1–4 Structural organization of the central and peripheral nervous systems.

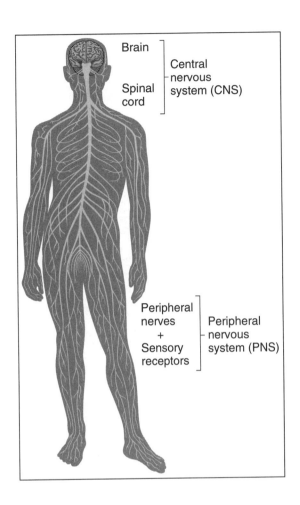

Brain

Spinal cord

Central nervous system (CNS)

Peripheral nerves + Sensory receptors

Peripheral nervous system (PNS)

The cardiovascular system in clients with diabetes is also greatly affected by the disease and is the cause of death in seventy percent of all clients diagnosed with the disease. Figure 1–5 shows the cardiovascular system. Hyperglycemia, hypoglycemia, and high levels of triglycerides all contribute to affects on the cardiovascular system. This system includes the heart, the arteries and veins, and all the peripheral vessels such as capillaries. The major affects on this system seen in clients with diabetes are myocardial infarction (MI), or heart attack, hypertension, and peripheral vascular disease. When circulation of the legs is poor, skin breakdown occurs, and ulcers may begin to appear. With continued hyperglycemia, these ulcers are difficult to heal.

The urinary system (see Figure 1–6) consists of the kidneys, bladder, urethra, and ureters. The urinary system is constantly challenged in hyperglycemic situations because as excess is spilled from the blood as waste, it attempts to rid the body of this unhealthy enemy. The combination of hypertension and glucose in the urine can lead to acute or chronic kidney disease in thirty to forty percent of insulin-dependent Diabetes Mellitus (IDDM) clients. In severe cases, these suffer from end stage renal disease and require kidney dialysis.

Figure 1–5 The Cardiovascular System.

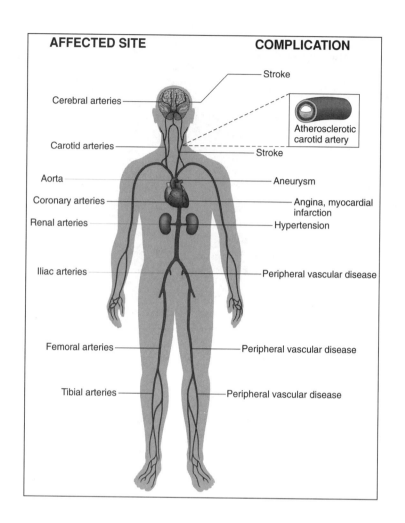

Figure 1–6 The Urinary System. (A) Posterior view of the kidneys, ureters, and bladder. (B) A nephron unit and related structures. Arrows indicate the flow of blood through the nephron.

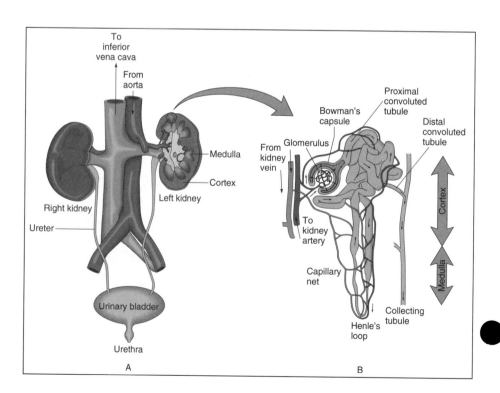

REVIEW QUESTIONS

1. The endocrine system regulates growth, reproduction, and _____ .

2. The _____ of _____ are small groups of cells in the pancreas.

3. Two hormones produced by the pancreas are _____ and _____ .

4. How many small groups of cells are located in the pancreas.

   a. one hundred

   b. one thousand

   c. ten thousand

   d. one million

5. Hormones are secreted directly into the

   a. pancreas

   b. kidney

   c. bloodstream

   d. tissue

6. The endocrine system includes

   a. ovaries and testes

   b. pituitary and adrenal glands

   c. pancreas

   d. all of the above

7. True or False? In diabetic clients, the pancreas usually produces enough insulin.

8. True or False? The circulatory system is not affected by diabetes.

10. Unscramble the following key term from this chapter: gaulcngo _____

CHAPTER 2

Overview of Diabetes

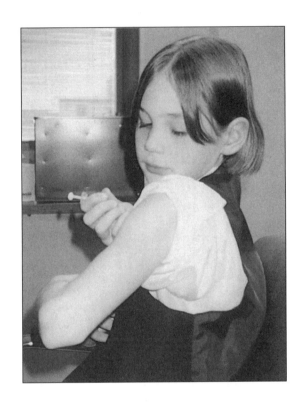

OBJECTIVES

Upon reading this chapter and completing the review questions, the home care aide should be able to:

1. Describe Diabetes Mellitus.
2. Describe physical changes seen in diabetic clients and explain why they occur.
3. Describe the signs and symptoms of diabetes.
4. Be familiar with the tests used to diagnose a client with diabetes.

KEY TERMS

complications
glucose
hyperglycemia
ketoacidosis
myocardial infarction (MI)

nephropathy
neuropathy
obesity
peripheral vascular disease (PVD)
retinopathy

INTRODUCTION

Diabetes Mellitus is one of the most common diseases seen by home health care personnel. It affects more than 14 million Americans and is the third leading cause of death by disease in the United States. Because this illness is chronic and has life-threatening complications, the client and their family require extensive care, particularly when the person is being treated at home. Diabetes Mellitus may be caused by **obesity** or pregnancy: but in these cases, it is not usually a permanent condition.

Diabetes results from a partial or complete lack of insulin, the hormone produced by the pancreas to convert sugar into energy. Insulin enables the body to store nutrients and metabolize carbohydrates and protein. If the client does not have enough insulin, the result is high blood sugar, or **hyperglycemia**. The diabetic client is treated by reducing carbohydrates and eliminating sugar in the diet, thereby regulating and balancing the insulin and blood sugar levels.

obesity the state of being overweight.

hyperglycemia high blood sugar.

TYPES OF DIABETES

It is important for HCAs to know the correct classification and type of diabetes of their client. Because diabetes is common among the elderly, health caregivers are constantly challenged to learn more about the disease. The specially trained HCA must be ready to assist the home health care team in meeting the needs of the diabetic client.

There are five main classifications of Diabetes. Each type is classified according to the age of the client, when the disease began, and the client's need for insulin. The types of diabetes are:

1. Diabetes Mellitus Type I, or Insulin-dependent (IDDM) Type I, occurs in 10 to 15 percent of all diabetes cases. This type is also called juvenile diabetes because it affects young persons before the age of 36. This form of diabetes may also be called brittle or familial diabetes. In this type, the body does not produce any insulin, and the client requires daily insulin injections for life. There are approximately 125,000 children in the United States with IDDM. Because the peak age of IDDM is 12 to 14 years in boys, and 10 to 12 years in girls, the onset may begin at puberty. Figure 2–1 shows a young girl with diabetes.

2. Diabetes Mellitus Type II, or non-insulin Dependent Diabetes (NIDDM) Type II, occurs in 85 percent to 90 percent of all diabetic cases, and usually involves adults over 36 years of age. In non-insulin dependent diabetics, the client either does not produce enough insulin, or produces enough insulin but which meets resistance at the receptor sites, causing it not to convert **glucose** (sugar) into the energy the body requires.

glucose natural sugar in foods.

NIDDM has a slow onset, and is generally the more stable type of the disease. It can be controlled with diet, exercise, and hypoglycemic drug therapy. This illness is most often seen in overweight women (especially black, Hispanic, and Native Americans) and the elderly.

3. Gestational Diabetes Type III occurs temporarily during pregnancy. The client returns to normal after delivery.

4. Diabetes Insipidus Type IV is a temporary condition caused by taking high doses of steroids or hormones. When the drugs are no longer taken, the diabetes disappears.

5. Diabetes Insidious Type V is a metabolic disorder caused by lack of antidiuretic hormone. In this type, the kidneys do not function properly. Mild cases are not usually treated, but drug therapy may be required in more serious cases.

NIDDM clients are seen in the home health setting, particularly where there are long-term effects of elevated glucose levels in elderly diabetic clients. Clients with Type I and II diabetes are commonly cared for in the home for unstable disease, diet training, and changes in medications. Diabetes in children is a challenge to both the health caregivers and the parents. Because

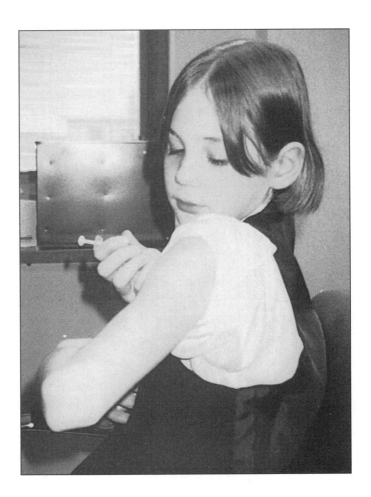

Figure 2–1 A young girl injects insulin into her arm.

complications a second disease, or abnormal condition occurring during the course of the primary disease.

both the body and weight change at a rapid rate, these young clients must be observed frequently and carefully for signs and symptoms of diabetic **complications**. Even very young diabetic children five or six years of age may care for themselves with the help and support of their caregivers and parents.

EFFECTS OF DIABETES

Physical changes commonly seen in clients with diabetes include eye, vascular, kidney, neurological, and skin problems. Diabetes is a chronic disease that is progressive, regardless of the cause or type. Insufficient levels of insulin lead to problems in the metabolism of carbohydrates, protein, and fat.

peripheral vascular disease (PVD) disease affecting the blood vessels.

retinopathy a disease affecting the retina of the eye.

nephropathy a disease affecting the kidneys.

neuropathy a disease affecting the nervous system.

Clients with diabetes have a higher risk for other chronic illnesses. The most common of these seen frequently in home health care setting are:

- cardiovascular disease
- **peripheral vascular disease (PVD)**
- **retinopathy**
- **nephropathy**
- **neuropathy**

Table 2–1 describes several complications of diabetes.

Table 2–1	**Complications of Diabetes**			
Long-Term Disorders	**Cause**	**Symptoms**	**Treatment**	**Aide's Care**
Blindness	Cataracts, glaucoma, hemorrhage	Partial or total loss of sight; client drops items; stumbles or falls; develops tunnel vision	Surgery can remove cataracts; medication or surgery for glaucoma	Assist in activities of daily living
Gangrene	Poor circulation; skin breakdown; invasion of tissue by bacteria	Heat in area, skin reddened, formation of ulcers which don't clear up; foul odor and spread of infection and tissue destruction	Medication under physician's order; may require amputation of limb	Assist with dressing changes and rehabilitation
Kidney disease	Too much sugar free in urine; filtering system works inefficiently	Frequency, pain, burning while voiding; retention of urine may occur	Diet modification and medication	Observe and record intake/output; note color and composition of urine
Vascular disease and nerve degeneration	High sugar level; poor fat metabolism; poor tissue repair; poor circulation	Open lesions form on skin tissue as vascular degeneration occurs; nervous system functions at decreased level; senses affected	Bed rest, moist heat dressings; diet and medication	Give proper foot care; assist in activities of daily living

In diabetes, glucose remains unchanged in the blood. Because of this, it builds up and affects the body in the following ways:

- fluids are out of balance because the kidneys are not functioning properly
- the immune system is suppressed
- circulation is impaired because of blood vessel restriction
- inadequate blood supply affects the brain, eyes, kidneys, and heart

Glucose, which provides the body with energy, is obtained primarily from dietary carbohydrates. Cells cannot use glucose without insulin which increases the transport of glucose through the cell membranes. In the client with diabetes, insulin is unavailable or unusable, and glucose remains in the bloodstream with some spilling into the urine.

In Type I diabetes (IDDM), the liver cannot handle the presence of glucose in the bloodstream, and excessive ketone bodies (a build-up of acetone as a result of the rapid breakdown of fat for energy) spill into the bloodstream. This is called **ketoacidosis**. In Type II diabetes (NIDDM), the limited insulin supply allows cells to function, but not at normal levels. In both situations, the client is in a dangerous and unstable condition until the physician diagnoses diabetes and orders treatment to stabilize the insulin and glucose.

ketoacidosis ketone bodies containing acetone spill into the bloodstream

SIGNS AND SYMPTOMS OF DIABETES

The classic signs and symptoms associated with Diabetes Mellitus usually come on slowly, but in some cases, appear quite suddenly. The signs and symptoms of diabetes include:

- polyuria (frequent urination with large amounts of urine output, and burning with urination)
- polydipsia (excessive thirst)
- polyphagia (excessive hunger)
- sudden and unusual weight loss
- itching
- weakness and irritability
- vaginitis (inflammation of the vagina)
- skin lesions and sores that heal slowly

The two most serious conditions that can arise in the diabetic client are **myocardial infarction** (MI) and peripheral vascular disease. The acute and chronic complications associated with diabetes are discussed in Chapters 5 and 6.

Helpful Hints: The HCA who cares for a client with diabetes in an unstable period must be specially trained to recognize sudden changes in the condition of the client.

myocardial infarction (MI) a heart attack

Helpful Hints: The prefix "poly" indicates excessive. The three "polys" identified above are important for specially trained HCAs to know.

DIAGNOSIS OF DIABETES

Diabetes Mellitus may be caused by the following factors:

- heredity
- obesity
- stress
- pregnancy, especially in mothers who deliver large babies (over 9 pounds)
- some medications such as steroids
- early onset of arterosclerotic heart disease
- chronic and recurring infections

Diagnosis of diabetes is made by a physician based on the results of the following five tests:

1. Fasting Blood Sugar (FBS)
2. Oral Glucose Tolerance Test (OGTT)
3. Two-hour Postpranial Glucose Test
4. Urinalysis for glycosuria or ketonuria
5. Glycosylated Hemoglobin AIC

Any or all of these tests may be ordered on diabetics cared for in the home setting. Unstable or uncontrolled diabetes is a commonly treated condition in home health. The HCA should be familiar with the types of laboratory tests that are indicated for the client, and the implications of abnormal test results.

The role of the HCA when such tests are ordered and included in Care Plan 1, may include all or some of the following:

1. Remove food and fluids at midnight or remind the client and/or family to do so if a test requires a period of fasting.
2. Assist the client to drink prescribed water or glucose drinks whenever and by what means they are ordered.
3. Assist the client/family to record results of home-based tests in a log for the nurse and the physician to review.
4. Collect urine samples as required, and encourage fluid intake when necessary. Store samples properly as the procedure states.
5. Assist the client in keeping track of when tests are to be done after eating meals or drinking glucose liquids.
6. Observe the client for unexpected symptoms when meals are served later than usual. Report these symptoms immediately.
7. If administering Clinitest or Acetests, keep accurate records and report any abnormal results to the supervisor.
8. Know test results, and when and if repeat tests are ordered; Place the date and time on the client's calendar.

Helpful Hints: Studies have shown that obesity contributes to increased incidence of diabetes in older adults.

Helpful Hints: It is important for HCAs to know when the client should or should not eat before certain tests.

The client must be educated about the tests the physician ordered because his or her understanding will affect the client's cooperation and responses to the treatment program.

IDENTIFICATION TAG

Because of the risk in emergency situations for clients with diabetes, it is important that he or she wears an identification tag or carries identification in the wallet or purse. Such identification alerts medical personnel that the wearer is a diabetic and could be in serious need of emergency treatment (see Figure 2–2)..

Clients with diabetes are often seen in home health care when the disease is newly diagnosed, the disease is suddenly unstable, or there are acute and severe chronic complications occurring because of the disease.

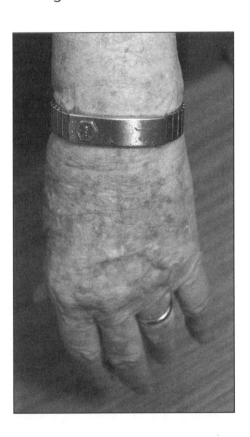

Figure 2–2 A Medic Alert® identification tag provides essential information in case of an emergency.

REVIEW QUESTIONS

1. Diabetes affects more than _____ million Americans.

2. The purpose of insulin is to convert _____ into energy.

3. a. IDDM is _____ _____ _____ _____.

   b. NIDDM is _____ _____ _____ _____ _____.

4. The three "polys" are:

   a.

   b.

   c.

5. Which of the following are types of diabetes?

   a. gestational

   b. juvenile

   c. insipidius

   d. all of the above

6. Which is not typical of NIDDM?

   a. it occurs in 90 percent of all cases

   b. it involves persons younger than 36

   c. clients do not produce enough insulin

   d. the body does not convert glucose

7. Most diabetic clients cared for in the home

   a. have unstable disease

   b. need diet training

   c. have changes in needs

   d. all of the above

8. True or False? Many elderly diabetics have eye changes to the retina.

9. True or False? Ketoacidosis is more common in Type II diabetes.

10. Unscramble the following key term from the chapter: hetunapoyr _____

Glucose Management and Control

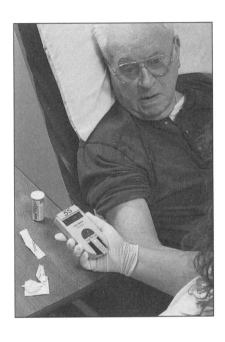

OBJECTIVES

Upon reading this chapter and completing the review questions, the home care aide should be able to:

1. Describe insulin therapy and the types and actions of insulin.

2. Describe hypoglycemia and insulin shock, and describe how to prevention them.

3. Be familiar with oral hypoglycemic agents, their actions, and indications.

4. Be familiar with glucose monitoring.

KEY TERMS

carbohydrate

glucose self-
 monitoring

hypoglycemia

insulin therapy

oral hypoglycemic agents (OHAs)

INTRODUCTION

When caring for diabetic clients, the most important concern is management of the glucose level. This is accomplished by the use of insulin, oral hypoglycemic agents, diet, exercise, or a combination. The HCA on the case should be familiar with these therapies, as well as glucose monitoring when assisting a diabetic client. This chapter focuses on the use of insulin and oral hypoglycemic agents to treat diabetes. Diet and exercise is discussed in Chapter 7.

INSULIN THERAPY

insulin therapy control of a diabetic patient with the use of insulin.

oral hypoglycemic agents (OHAs) oral medications that boost the pancreas to produce insulin.

When hyperglycemia occurs in diabetes, insulin from another source must be provided. The treatment of diabetes with insulin is called **insulin therapy**. This can be in the form of **oral hypoglycemic agents (OHAs)** or injectable insulin. Since the 1980s, oral hypoglycemic agents have been successful with close supervision for insulin regulation. The insulin duration (how long the coverage lasts) varies with the type of insulin or OHA agent, but most are 10 to 16 hours, 12 to 24 hours, and 10 to 20 hours.

Home health aides do not give insulin injections. However, specially trained HCAs may be asked to obtain the bottle from the refrigerator and gather the supplies to assist the client. The date on the insulin must not have expired for it to be safe for client use. The client is taught by the nurse to carefully measure the dose in a syringe and to use sterile technique for drawing and injecting the insulin (see Figure 3–1). Specially trained HCAs should know that the insulin must be taken at the same prescribed time every day.

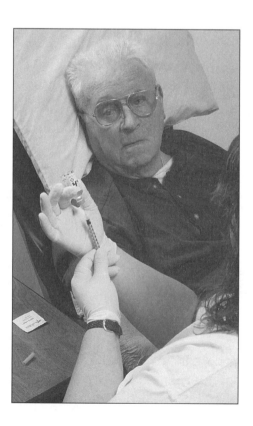

Figure 3–1 The nurse teaches the client how to inject himself with insulin.

Helpful Hints: If the injection site appears red or warm to the touch, the HCA should call the nurse or supervisor immediately.

Most clients use their abdomen, upper arms, and thighs for sites of injection, and are taught to change the site frequently. Figure 3–2 shows the possible sites for insulin injection. The HCA might see evidence of recent injections on these areas when providing personal care of the client.

Insulin pumps may be used by some diabetic clients. A small needle is placed in the abdomen and connected to a pump worn at the client's waist. The client controls the amount of insulin entering the body by pressing a button. The nurse will teach the client and the family how to use and maintain the pump when it is prescribed by the physician.

For uncontrolled diabetes, injection is the usual method of treatment. Figure 3–3 shows a young girl injecting insulin into her arm. Insulin that is injected into muscle acts slowly and reaches the bloodstream in one dose which is unlike insulin that is produced by the body in response to ingested food. The physician determines the type of insulin based on the results of blood tests, diet, urine tests, and information from the nurse such as the activity level of the client. There are slow-acting, intermediate-acting, and rapid-acting types of insulin. The specially trained HCA must be familiar with all types of insulin, and their peak action and duration (see Table 3–1).

Table 3–1 Types of Insulin		
Type of Insulin	**Peak Actiion**	**Length of Action**
Rapid Acting (Regular, Semilente)	3–4 hours	6–8 hours
Intermediate (Lente, NPH, Globulin)	9 hours	24 hours
Slow Acting (PZI, Ultralente)	20 hours	36 hours

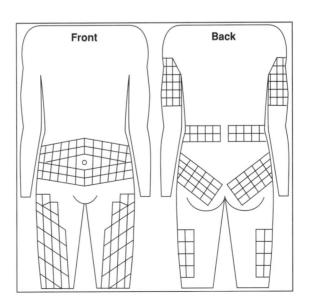

Figure 3–2 The areas of the body where insulin can be injected.

Figure 3–3 A little girl injects insulin into her arm.

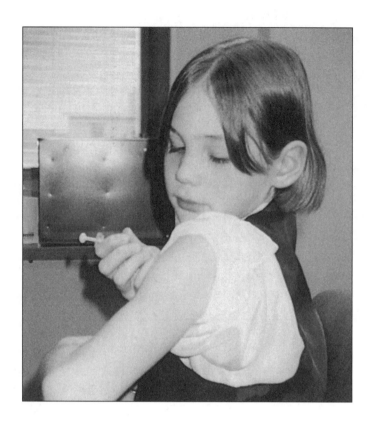

Helpful Hints: The HCA who has knowledge of insulin actions and durations will understand the importance of observing clients for insulin instability.

carbohydrates compounds of carbons, hydrogens, and oxygen, such as sugars and starches; most are formed by green plants.

hypoglycemia low blood sugar.

The major action of insulin is to lower blood sugar by allowing glucose to enter the cells for storage as glycogen or burned for energy. If glucose cannot enter cells because of a lack of insulin, it is excreted in the urine. Normal fasting blood sugar (FBS), the blood sugar level when the client has not eaten, is usually 70–110 mg/dl. Levels of 140 mg/dl or greater obtained on two or more occasions, confirm the diagnosis of Diabetes Mellitus if other causes have been ruled out.

Blood glucose regulation is the primary goal of caring for diabetic client in home care. It is important for the HCA to understand glucose metabolism. Glucose is used as the basic energy source by the body, and it is important that the level be in balance. Hormones and enzymes maintain balance in the body by helping the body to use (metabolize) glucose for energy. The most important of these is glucagon, which causes blood sugar levels to rise by converting stored sugar (glycogen) to glucose and insulin.

When the body cannot use **carbohydrates** efficiently, it metabolizes fat, and ketone bodies show up in the blood and urine. Excess amounts of insulin in the bloodstream lead to **hypoglycemia**, a decreased level of glucose concentration in the blood. Hypoglycemia occurs when the client exercises, has a high protein intake, or has increased stress because of the higher rate of use of the available glycogen. This causes initial symptoms of irritability, sweating, and hunger. If left untreated, the client experiences giddiness, coma and death.

Abnormal carbohydrate, fat, and protein metabolism causes an increase in blood glucose levels (hyperglycemia). The client with hyperglycemia will show the following signs and symptoms:

- increased thirst
- loss of appetite
- labored breathing
- sweet or fruity odor of breath
- frequent urination
- severe weight loss
- poor skin texture
- sunken eyes
- dry mouth and cracked lips

Observation and reporting of insulin therapy is an on-going process during the course of the treatment of the diabetic client in home care. The client and family's cooperation in this area will vary, depending on their ability to understand and apply insulin therapy.

ORAL HYPOGLYCEMIC AGENTS

Helpful Hints: Remember, these drugs are not for Type I diabetics who are on injectable insulin.

In persons with NIDDM, the disease is often controlled by diet. Occasionally, oral hypoglycemic agents (OHAs), called sulfonylureas, are ordered in pill form as well. These medications stimulate the client's endogenous production of insulin. Close medical supervision is necessary for dosage regulation, and the HCA may be involved in observing the client for signs and symptoms of an insulin imbalance.

Clients most likely to respond well to OHAs are those who:

- had onset of hyperglycemia after age 30
- have had diagnosed hyperglycemia for more than five years
- are of normal weight or who are obese
- are willing to follow a diet regimen
- are not insulin dependent

The HCA's duty in caring for clients with diabetes who are on OHAs is to observe if the client is taking the medication regularly, and reporting to the supervisor if the client is not (see Figure 3–4). The client with diabetes who has been placed on OHAs in home health has been placed on a new medication. Therefore, the skilled nurse will teach the client and the family about the side effects and uses of this medication. Because the medication has to be adjusted to each client's condition, diet, and exercise level, it is important for the HCA to observe and report any unusual reactions or condition changes during this initial period of

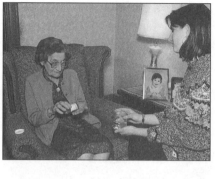

Figure 3–4 The HCA observes if the client takes her medication regularly, and reports to the supervisor if the client does not.

the body's adjustment. Any questions the client might have should be communicated to the nurse or supervisor on the case so the physician and the nurse can discuss them with the family and the client. Some OHAs are taken before breakfast and the evening meal; others are taken with breakfast or the first main meal of the day. Still others are taken 30 minutes before breakfast. Healthcare givers who assist the client with medications must follow the care plan to ensure that medications are given at the proper times prescribed by the physician.

Combination insulin therapy usually includes a dosage plan with two types of insulin, such as regular OHAs in the morning and injectible insulin at bedtime. Such combination therapy with both injectable insulin and OHAs is still being tested. Most common is a bedtime injection of intermediate insulin with a daytime OHA. This new combination therapy requires careful blood glucose and urine glucose monitoring until the client is stabilized on the dosage.

Newly ordered OHAs may have to be increased or decreased in dosage during the first few weeks of treatment. The urine and blood will be tested for glucose frequently during this period. It is important that a log be kept by the client, the family, or the HCA with the results of the tests recorded over a specific period of time. This log may be the determining factor upon which the physician bases a change of dosage. It is also important that the client's diet be carefully observed, as well as his or her activity and exercise level.

Common problems associated with the use of OHAs are:

- hypoglycemia
- gastrointestinal disturbances
- allergic reactions
- water retention
- low sodium levels in the blood
- lower-than-normal blood platelets resulting in bleeding and bruising
- jaundice
- interactions with other drugs

Helpful Hints: The HCA and the family should keep a log, and carefully record the client's response to new insulin therapy programs.

GLUCOSE MONITORING

In the 1970s, capillary blood glucose testing began in the home, but was complicated and expensive. Today, modern devices are inexpensive, accurate, and easy to use (see Figure 3–5). In addition, **glucose self-monitoring** is practical, and offers a comprehensive overview of the client's glucose levels over a 24-hour period, showing clearly the effects of insulin, food, stress, diet, and exercise in relation to the glucose level.

Many new products are available and most are purchased with excellent written, audio or video instructions. The best finger sticking devices are spring controlled and puncture only as deep as necessary to get the drop of blood required to do the test. Figure 3–6 shows a finger sticking device. The specialty trained HCA should first study glucose monitoring information so he can answer accurately any questions the client may have about the operation and cleaning of the equipment.

The number of times per day blood glucose should be monitored is dependent on the following factors:

- the physician's order
- the stability of insulin therapy
- the stability of blood glucose levels
- nocturnal hypoglycemia
- periods of illness
- stability of diet management
- periods of stress
- exercise changes

Glucose monitoring is important for clients with newly diagnosed diabetes in order for the physician to evaluate the treatment plan prescribed. In addition, for those diabetics who are experiencing a period of instability, glucose monitoring is important in order for the physician to determine if a change in the prescribed insulin therapy is needed. All chronic diabetics do glucose monitoring daily to ensure that their glucose levels are under control.

glucose self-monitoring   the client learns to do glucose testing himself on an easy to use device at home.

Helpful Hints: The nurse will teach the diabetic client how to do glucose self-monitoring, and more important, when to call the physician to report unusual results. It is the responsibility of the HCA to reinforce the nurse's teachings.

Helpful Hints: The Department of Health regulations for the HCA's state may require the nurse to do on-site instruction to the HCA for each client they care for in order to assure the competence of the care given.

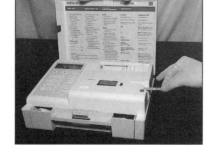

Figure 3–5   By placing one drop of blood on a special stick, this machine shows the blood sugar level in about one minute.

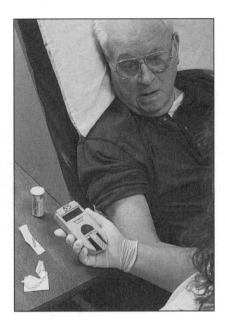

Figure 3–6 This shows a finger-stick device used to monitor the client's glucose level.

Three new methods of insulin administration come in a nasal spray, eye drops, and programmable, implantable medication systems (PIMs) such as a pump unit placed in the abdomen which has a five-year battery and a hand-held radio transmitter to control insulin release.

REVIEW QUESTIONS

1. Two sources of insulin production outside of the pancreas are _____ and _____ .

2. Slow-acting PZI insulin reaches its peak action at _____ .

3. Rapid-acting insulin is also called _____ .

4. Which of the following is not a type of insulin?
   a. ultralente
   b. NPH
   c. Extremely slow acting
   d. Rapid acting

5. Normal FBS is
   a. 70–110
   b. 70–120
   c. 110–140
   d. 110–160

6.Which is not a contributing factor of insulin shock?

    a. stress

    b. diet

    c. exercise

    d. hyperglycemia

7.Clients most likely to respond well to OHAs are

    a. of normal weight

    b. not insulin dependent

    c. experienced onset after age 30

    d. all of the above

8. True or False? OHAs are not considered medications.

9. True or False? Most diabetics can do glucose self-monitoring.

10. Unscramble the following key term from the chapter: ypoghycmieal _____

CHAPTER 4

HCA Roles and Functions

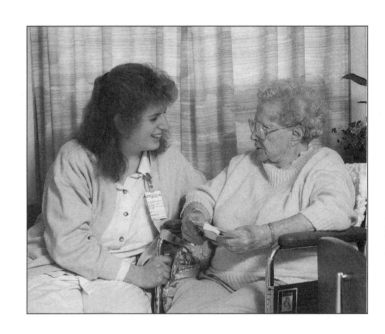

OBJECTIVES

Upon reading this chapter and completing the review questions, the home care aide should be able to:

1. Describe the home health care aide's responsibilities of observing and reporting when caring for the client with diabetes.

2. Describe observation of the clients body by body system.

3. Describe twelve areas that should be addressed by the HCA when caring for a client with diabetes.

4. Define and describe documentation, including general guidelines.

5. Be familiar with the HCA care plan, and the HCA's roles, responsibilities, and functions when caring for a client with diabetes.

KEY TERMS

documentation
HCA care plan

limitations
palpitations

INTRODUCTION

The roles and functions of the specially trained HCA are varied. While providing personal care, nutrition management, and home maintenance for their clients, HCAs must be skillful in observing, reporting, and documentating. In addition, they must understand the HCA care plan as it relates to the care of the client with diabetes.

OBSERVATION AND REPORTING

Observation and reporting are skills expected of the HCA. A specially trained HCA is expected to have even greater skills in the area of observation, reporting, and **documentation** of the client with diabetes. Some of the questions the HCA should ask during the visit include the following:

documenation the written account of what is seen, heard, and observed by the HCA.

* Have there been any changes in the client's level of energy?
* Have there been changes in the client's ability to perform activities of daily living?
* Has the client's family noticed any changes in mental status, such as increased forgetfulness?
* Has there been an increase in the loss of patience with self or others?
* Has the client felt more irritable, nervous, or anxious?
* Does the client complain of fatigue, numbness, or tingling in the feet and hands?
* Is the client experiencing pain, such as headaches, bone pain, or abdominal pain?
* Has the client complained of nausea or loss of appetite?

palpitations excessive pounding of the heart.

* Does the client experience any **palpitations** (excessive pounding of the heart), shortness of breath, or dizziness?

The HCA must report all changes in the client's condition to the nurse or supervisor. Figure 4–1 shows an HCA asking the client with diabetes questions on her visit.

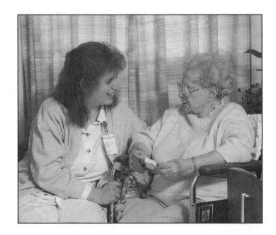

Figure 4–1 The HCA asks the client questions during her visit, and reports all changes in the client's condition to the nurse or supervisor.

Physical Observations

The nurse's physical exam includes the gathering of important information about the client's body. Once the initial physical exam has been performed, the HCA should observe the following on each visit:

- the physical appearances of the client's skin for dryness, scars, bruising, swelling, excessive perspiration, elevated temperature, or open or reddened areas
- brittleness of the nails
- the lower extremities for poor circulation and loss of sensation in the feet which leads to skin breakdown and ulcers
- the extremities for weakness, walking problems, twitching, balance problems, tremors, or spasms
- the feet for color, skin condition, ulcers, warmth or coolness of the skin, calluses, and thickened nails
- changes in the gastrointestinal function including polyphagia, polydipsia, appetite changes, mouth and tongue sores, vomiting, diarrhea, constipation, dehydration, weight changes, or obesity
- changes in the urinary function such as voiding problems, incontinence, pain when voiding, or blood in the urine
- general changes such as moods, vital signs, activity level, nutrition, and hydration
- changes in breathing, cough, and nasal or chest congestion.

The HCA should observe the client on each visit and report the appearance of any of these signs and symptoms. Some information will be obtained from family members or friends who often play significant roles. Questions for family members or friends include:

- Is the client slowed, inactive, depressed, or behaving out of the ordinary?
- Are there changes in consciousness such as drowsiness, slow thinking, inappropriate responses to questions, or confusion?

Many times, the family will relate important information to the HCA during the visit, and any changes in the client's condition must be reported immediately to the supervisor.

Twelve Areas of Concern

If the client is a known diabetic, the following twelve areas should be observed by the HCA during visits and results reported to the supervisor or nurse on the case:

1. excessive urination
2. excessive thirst

3. excessive hunger

4. weight loss or gain

5. blurred vision

6. burning sensation when urinating

7. infections

8. injuries

9. medications not taken

10. skipped meals or uneaten food

11. reddened injection sites

12. itching

> **Helpful Hints:** If the client expresses a problem, the HCA should determine if this is a new problem and if not, has it been treated before and how it was treated.

Before reporting observations and/or changes to the supervisor, the HCA should always:

1. Gather all possible information first.

2. Check the client's vital signs.

3. Know the agency's or facility's policies on reporting patient information.

When reporting on the telephone, the HCA should begin with his or her name and the name of the client. If a telephone message is left, the HCA should give the date, time, telephone number, and a description of the situation. The HCA must document everything observed and report it on the visit form. Figure 4–2 shows an HCA documenting her observations. Careful observation and reporting is vital when caring for a client with diabetes. The HCA is the health caregiver in the home and at the bedside most frequently, and his or her eyes and ears gather important information for the other members of the home care team.

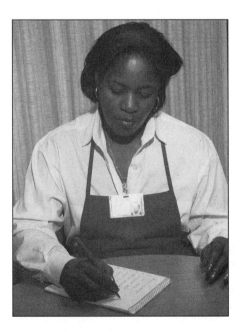

Figure 4–2 Careful observation and reporting is vital when caring for a client with diabetes.

DOCUMENTATION

Documentation is the written record of the HCA's observations and reporting. Objective documentation is the recording of signs that are seen, heard, smelt, or felt. The proper documentation style for recording signs is to write a sentence or statement such as: the patient's skin is moist and cool, and the color is white and pale.

Subjective documentation is the recording of symptoms, or what the client says. The proper documentation style is to place the client's statement in quotations, such as, the client states "I am having a lot of burning and pain when I urinate."

The written documentation becomes part of the client's permanent record which is a legal document. It is proof that the HCA made the visit, and which tasks have been performed. The specially trained HCA should write each note as if the physician, the insurance company, or the court system will be reading it in the future.

Specially trained HCAs should also have an increased vocabulary in the area chosen. They are expected to communicate and document at a level higher than that of other HCAs. It is important for them to study the new terms in this module and make them part of their daily reporting and recording.

The following are guidelines for documentation:

Helpful Hints: Agencies have a rule stating, "If it was not documented, it was not done." This means that documentation is the only proof of the care given.

- The client record is written evidence of the care given, the patient's response, and the outcome of the care.

- The client record reflects changes in orders so that all members of the health care team are kept current.

- The client record is a communication tool on which the plan for care is outlined.

- The client record is a written document required by insurance companies and regulatory agencies.

- The client record may be used in a court to prove that care was given, observations were documented, or as evidence for court-ordered guardians or vulnerable adults.

- Recording should be descriptive, with a note about each complaint or problem.

- Use words that are descriptive rather than general terms such as "normal" or "good."

- Writing should be neat.

- Recording should be done in black ink.

- Recording should begin with the date and time, and end with a signature and title.

- Recording should include the time a change was noticed, and in long-term cases, a note at least every two hours.

- When quoting client symptoms, use quotation marks.
- All attempts to report to the supervisor should be carefully documented. If a message is left, it should be written on the record with whom they spoke, the date, and the time.
- Errors should not be erased; instead, a line should be drawn through the wrong entry and initials placed next to it.
- Only abbreviations accepted by the agency should be used.
- HCAs should chart observations and activities that are their own.
- Their signature legally states that they completed the procedure and documented it.
- If a new page is added, the client's name must be on each new page, and the time and date written again.
- HCAs should not skip lines when writing documentation, sign all visit forms, and leave no spaces between the notes and the signature.

HCA CARE PLAN

HCA Care Plan the plan written by the nurse-in-charge specifying the care to be provided by the HCA on each client visit.

The **HCA care plan** for the client with diabetes will be determined by the nurse on the case. The Specific Treatment and Instructions section can be adapted to the client with diabetes. The nurse can then make the HCA care plan individualized for that particular client, based on the nursing diagnoses, goals, and expected outcomes. As the client's condition progresses or changes, the nurse will continually update the care plan in the Changes section of the form.

The HCA care plan is divided into eight main sections that the HCA should include on any single visit (see Figure 4–3). These include:

Helpful Hints: The HCA's role in caring for the client is reflected in the care plan. The HCA should not perform any procedures that are not defined in the care plan.

- personal care
- nutrition
- bowel and bladder elimination
- activity
- safety precautions
- family member(s)
- mental status

limitations restriction of activity.

- **limitations**

The HCA care plan contains, in addition to these routine areas of concern, care areas specific to the client with diabetes and would most likely include the following:

- medical nutrition
- insulin management control

BOSTON REGIONAL MEDICAL CENTER/HEALTH CARE AT HOME

Home Health Aide Assignment

Client Name: _____ I.D.#: _____

Address: _____ Telephone#: (____)____ - ____

Contact Person: _____ Telephone#: (____)____ - ____

Directions to Home: _____

Diagnosis: _____ Age: _____

Fee Source: _____

Other Disciplines Following:

____ HHA   ____ R.N.   ____ P.T.   ____ O.T.   ____ S.T.   ____ S.W.

Patient Status:

Mental Status:	Incontinence:	Toileting:	Impairments:	Mobility Aids:	Activities:
—Alert	—Bowel	—Bedpan	—Speech	—Cane	—Ambulatory
—Forgetful	—Bladder	—Commode	—Hearing	—Walker	—Amb w/Ass't.
—Confused		—Bathroom	—Vision	—Crutches	—Bed Bound
—Depressed		—Catheter	—Sensation	—W/C	—W/C Bound
		—Urinal	—Paralysis	—Prosthesis	
			—Contracture	—Other	
			—Amputation		
			—Decubiti		

ASSIGNMENT: Check or circle appropriate items. Indicate frequency of assignment (eg: pm; 1 x wk; etc.)

PERSONAL CARE:	NUTRITION:	SPECIAL SERVICES:
☐ Bath-sponge	☐ Special Diet	☐ Exercise if requested by PT/RN
☐ Bath-Tub/Shower	☐ Meal Preparation	☐ Ambulation-Walker, etc.
☐ Bath-Partial	☐ Encourage Fluids	☐ Special Skin Care
☐ Hair-Shampoo/Grooming	☐ Feeding/Serving	☐ Weigh Patient
☐ Nails and/or Shave		☐ Measure intake/output
☐ Mouth Care	HOUSEHOLD: Marketing	☐ Check bowel elimination
☐ Bed Making	☐ Laundry	☐ Assist with Medication
☐ Help with Dressing	☐ Care of Bedroom	☐ Accompany to M.D.
☐ Help with Toileting	☐ Care of Kitchen	☐ Pulse, Respiration and B.P.
☐ Transfer to Wheelchair	☐ Care of Bathroom	☐ Temperature-Oral/Axillary
☐ Turn every—hours	☐ Care of Living Room	☐ Dressing Change/Wound Care
☐ Lotion/Massage	☐ Linen Change	☐ Ostomy Care
☐	☐ Light Housework	☐ Catheter Care/Empty Drainage Bag
☐	☐	☐

BP:_____   Pulse: _____

Other:_____

ADDITIONAL INSTRUCTIONS/SAFETY PRECAUTIONS:

_____

_____

_____

_____

_____

Signature of Nurse/Therapist: _____   Date: _____

Freq/Visits: _____   Preference of Days: ____   Time: ____ AM ____ PM

Case Manager: Primary HHA: _____   Date: _____

Signature of Assigned Personnel: _____

ASSIGNMENT REVIEW:

Date: _____	Initials: _____	Date: _____	Initials: _____
Date: _____	Initials: _____	Date: _____	Initials: _____
Date: _____	Initials: _____	Date: _____	Initials: _____

EMERGENCY NUMBERS:

Distribution:	Yellow	—	Chart
	Pink	—	HHA
	Green	—	Patient's Home

Figure 4–3 An example of a Home Care Aide care plan that lists the assigned duties (Courtesy Boston Regional Medical Center/Health Care at Home, Stoneham, MA).

- infection prevention
- exercise management
- glucose monitoring
- self-care techniques
- oral hypoglycemic agents
- foot care

In order to accommodate the increased activities on the HCA care plan, appropriate documentation is necessary for the HCA care plan to be specific to the client with diabetes. Figure 4–4 is an example of a Visit Form specifically designed to guide the HCA to consider these specific activities at each visit. Observation and reporting are expected on each HCA visit, but some procedures specific for diabetic care will be performed on some clients and not on others. Therefore, the care plan is divided into those routine tasks that should be done on every visit and those which the nurse will instruct the specially trained HCA to do for that specific client on that visit. Each agency has forms utilized specifically and the HCA must be familiar with all of them.

HOME CARE AIDE ROLES AND FUNCTIONS

As the HCA is given more responsibility in the home care field, the nurse and the HCA will become a closely working team based on the following two important aspects: communication and coordination. Often, all members of the care team meet to discuss the client's progress (see Figure 4–5).

In the future, the HCA's roles and functions will increase and become more specific to caring for clients with unique problems. For this training module in caring for diabetic clients, the new roles and functions of the HCA include:

- having a knowledge of the signs of insulin shock and diabetic coma, and to report them immediately to the supervisor
- knowing the emergency treatment for mild hypoglycemia
- being knowledgeable about insulin therapy, observing and evaluating the client for signs and symptoms of insulin imbalance, and reporting any changes to the supervisor as quickly as possible
- being aware of the importance of proper diet management, and observing and evaluating the client's nutrition level, particularly his or her noncompliance and/or foods on the diet plan uneaten by the client
- being knowledgeable concerning foot care, prevention of complications, and the reporting of any problem areas to the supervisor

Health Education Inc. Home Care Aide Visit Form for Diabetes

Name _____ No: _____ Diagnosis: _____
Home Care Aide: _____ Date of visit: _____
Date of Discharge: _____ Nurse: _____

Routine Care:	Date:	Documentation:	Sign:
I. Observe Extremities			
A. Temperature			
B. Color			
C. Numbness			
D. Pain			
E. Ulcerations			
F. Tingling			
II. Observe and Evaluate Skin			
A. Itching			
B. Burning			
C. Positioning for pressure points			
D. Ulcerations			
E. Wound			
III. Observe Diet and Food Intake			
A. Glucometer			
B. Urine testing			
C. S&S hyperglycemia			
D. S&S hypoglycemia			
IV. Observeand Evaluate Ambulation			
A. Safety pecautions			
B. Visual problems			
C. Unsteady gait			
D. Assisting devices			
E. Environment			
V. Observe and Evaluate Infection (S&S)			
A. TPR			
B. Redden warm area			
C. Chills			
D. Infection control			
E. Wound drainage			
VI. Observeand Evaluate Exercise/Activity Level			
A. Physical exercise as ordered			
B. Physical exercise *not* ordered			
C. Decrease in exercise as ordered			
D. ROM			
VII. Observe and Evaluate Elimination			
A. Incontinent			
B. Constipation			
C. Diarrhea			
D. Urine clear			
E. Urine cloudy, dark			
F. Frequency/Burning on urination			
G. Excessive perspiraiton			
H. Adequate/inadequate fluid intake			
IX. Observe and Evaluate Mental Status			
A. Depression			
B. Confusion			
C. Forgetfulness			
D. State of agitation			
E. Stress			
F. Oriented			

Specific Treatments/Procedures:	Date:	Documentation:	Sign:
Skin Care			
Decubitus Care			
Prevention of Joint Deformities			
Dietary: Intake Logging I&O			
Glucometer			
Clinitest			
Acetest			
Bladder Training			

Figure 4–4 An example of a Visit Form specifically designed to guide the HCA to consider specific activites at each visit. (Courtesy Health Education, Inc.)

- testing urine for the presence of glucose and/or ketones
- being aware of the importance of proper skin care

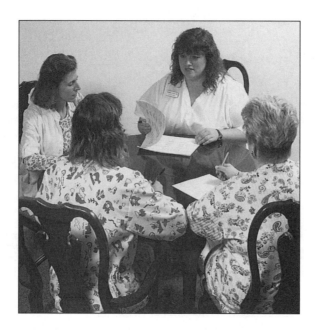

Figure 4–5 All members are an important part of the care team and may often meet to discuss the client's progress.

Helpful Hints: Specially trained HCAs who are caring for clients with diabetes must keep current on diabetic care by reading and taking inservice courses on diabetes at regular intervals.

- observing and evaluating the skin, and reporting any problem areas to the supervisor
- being knowledgeable about glucose monitoring
- being aware of acute and chronic complications of the client with diabetes, observing for signs and symptoms, and reporting any problem areas to the supervisor

The one important function of the HCA caring for a client with diabetes that will be increasing is documentation. Documentation has always been a responsibility of the HCA, particularly in the recording of changes in the client. However, in the specialization of care of the client with diabetes, more documentation is necessary as proof of the services provided by the HCA to the client and observations of that client by the HCA.

REVIEW QUESTIONS

1. Before reporting observations or changes to the supervisor, the HCA should:
    a. gather _____
    b. check _____
    c. know _____
2. _____ is the written record of observations and reporting.
3. a. Symptoms are _____
    b. Signs are _____

4. Which of the following are physical observations of the skin?
   a. dryness
   b. coolness
   c. burning
   d. tingling
5. Which are signs or symptoms that should be reported?
   a. irritability
   b. loss of energy
   c. headache
   d. all of the above
6. Legs should be observed for
   a. weakness
   b. twitching
   c. poor circulation
   d. all of the above
7. Which is not one of the twelve observable concerns specific in care of the diabetic?
   a. injuries
   b. family relationships
   c. infections
   d. excessive thirst
8. True or False? Weight gain or loss should be a concern in the client with diabetes
9. True or False? The HCA care plan is written by the HCA.
10. Unscramble the following key term from the chapter: tnidetocuamon _____

Acute Complications

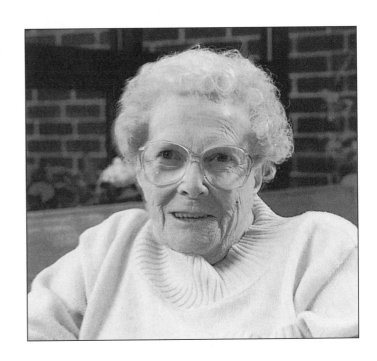

OBJECTIVES

Upon reading this chapter and completing the review questions, the home care aide should be able to:

1. Describe four acute complications of diabetes.
2. Describe the symptoms of hypoglycemia.
3. Describe the symptoms of hyperglycemia.
4. Describe the symptoms of insulin shock.

KEY TERMS

acute   **insulin shock**

hypoglycemic coma

INTRODUCTION

Clients with diabetes are often seen in the home health setting with acute complications which must be treated, but do not require an admission to a hospital or skilled nursing facility. In addition, unstable or new diabetics seen in the home must be observed closely for signs and symptoms of acute complications.

acute severe, but of short duration.

Therefore, it is important for the specially trained HCA to be familiar with the acute complications of diabetes.

The following are **acute** complications of diabetes:

- Hypoglycemia
- Hyperglycemia
- Ketoacidosis
- Hyperglycemic Coma
- Insulin Shock

HYPOGLYCEMIA

hypoglycemic coma a condition caused by low levels of sugar in the bloodstream.

Hypoglycemia is a low level of sugar in the bloodstream. The signs and symptoms associated with **hypoglycemia** include:

- excessive perspiration
- faintness, dizziness, weakness
- nervousness
- hunger; numbness of tongue and lips
- irritability
- altered level of consciousness (such as coma or unconsciousness)
- headache
- blurred vision
- tremors
- staggering gait
- pale, moist skin

The HCA should contact the nursing supervisor if the client has any of these symptoms, and should always document what he or she sees. The HCA may be required to give the client a concentrated dose of sugar if any of these symptoms occur. Examples of foods that may be used for hypoglycemic episodes include:

For 10 grams of carbohydrates:

- 4 life savers
- 4 ounces of orange juice
- 4 ounces of nondietetic soda
- 2 teaspoons of honey
- 2 teaspoons of sugar

For 15 grams of carbohydrates:

- 6 saltines
- 8 unces of nondietetic soda
- 4 ounces of apple juice
- 6 vanilla wafers
- 2 graham crackers

Helpful Hints: The HCA must have a specific order from the physician as to what foods or sugar doses are appropriate for each diabetic client.

KETOACIDOSIS

Ketones are the products of fat metabolism in hyperglycemia. They spill into the urine along with excess sugar, causing ketonuria which can be monitored by testing the urine. A high concentration of ketone bodies can result in diabetic coma. Figure 5–1 shows the differences between ketoacidosis and acute hypoglycemia. Ketosis is the increase of ketones in the blood, and usually occurs over a 24-hour period in response to a sudden need for insulin brought on by stress, illness, infection, injury, or sudden inactivity. The client is in a dangerous and unstable condition until the physician diagnoses diabetes and orders treatment to stabilize the insulin and glucose levels. The signs and symptoms of diabetic ketoacidosis (DKA) occur from the changes in body fluid and include some or all of the following:

- polyuria
- polyphagia
- fatigue and eye weakness
- headache
- muscle aches
- abdominal pain
- nausea, vomiting; other stomach symptoms
- fever, if infection is present
- increased respiratory rate, air hunger
- sweetish (fruity) odor on breath due to acidemia
- drowsy to comatose

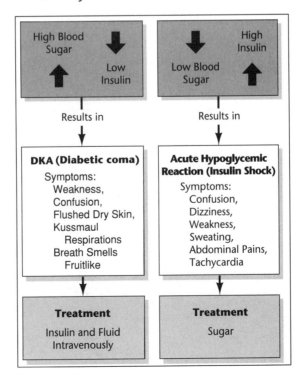

Figure 5–1 Difference between ketoacidosis and acute hypoglycemia.

If the client with diabetes appears to be in a ketoacidotic state, the HCA should call 911 first, then the supervisor. Document every detail observed. Emergency treatment is to quickly restore balance in the client's blood glucose level and electrolytes. Figure 5–2 shows a client exhibiting symptoms of a ketoacidotic coma. The HCA should take vital signs and continue to monitor them until emergency measures are taken. The HCA may be asked to meet the ambulance and to give the responders a short history of the client's status. This includes any evidence of recent infection, noncompliance to insulin prescription or diet program, and any other possible causes for the ketoacidosis.

HYPERGLYCEMIA

Hyperglycemia occurs when there are large amounts of sugar in the bloodstream. The signs and symptoms associated with hyperglycemia include:

- increased respiration
- labored breathing
- loss of appetite
- nausea and/or vomiting
- weakness
- abdominal pains
- generalized ache
- increased thirst
- sweet or fruity odor on the breath
- flushed, dry skin
- loss of consciousness or confusion
- polyuria

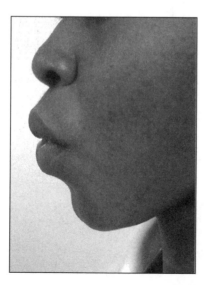

Figure 5–2 A client exhibits symptoms of a ketoacidotic coma. The client's lips are pressed together and her respirations are deep and rapid.

Helpful Hints: Any HCA caring for a diabetic client with high levels of blood glucose should check vital signs, urine glucose if possible, and call the supervisor quickly.

A client in a hyperglycemic state has blood glucose levels ranging from 300 to 1800 mg/dl.

When caring for clients with infections, insulin dosages must never be lowered because of loss of appetite. The physician should be notified immediately, and frequent glucose monitoring done during this time.

Hyperglycemic coma is an emergency situation which calls for immediate measures to stabilize the blood glucose level. This may occur in:

- an acute illness such as pneumonia, MI, or CVA
- a drug reaction to insulin instability
- therapeutic procedures such as kidney dialysis or Total Parental Nutrition (TPN) which is admistration of sterile liquid protien directly into the blood stream.

The causes of a hyperglycemic coma include:

- insufficient insulin
- overeating
- undiagnosed diabetes
- lack of exercise
- stress as a result of illness, infection, surgery, or emotional problems

The signs and symptoms of hyperglycemic coma include:

- weakness
- drowsiness
- thirst
- hunger
- sweet, fruity odor on the breath
- flushed cheeks
- slow, deep, and labored respirations
- low blood pressure
- dry skin
- headache
- nausea and vomiting
- coma

If the client is in a hyperglycemic coma, it is vital to call 911 immediately, take the vital signs, and stay with the client. If possible, call the supervisor so that the physician can be contacted for emergency orders. If this is not possible, the client should be taken to the emergency room. The mortality rate of a hyperglycemic coma is 5 percent to 50 percent depending on the severity of the symptoms.

The complications associated with hyperglycemic coma include:

- hypotension (low blood pressure)
- dehydration (dry mucous membranes, dry skin)
- fever
- tachycardia (rapid heart rate)
- seizures and/or coma

INSULIN SHOCK

insulin shock shock as a result of excessive amounts of insulin in the blood

The causes of **insulin shock** include:

- excessive amounts of insulin
- omitting a meal
- inadequate food intake
- excessive physical activity
- vomiting

The signs and symptoms of insulin shock include:

- hunger
- weakness
- trembling
- dizziness
- headache
- perspiration
- rapid pulse
- low blood pressure
- cold, clammy skin (diaphoresis)
- confusion, irritability and personality changes
- convulsion
- unconsciousness

If the client with diabetes has any of these signs and symptoms, the HCA must call 911 immediately, take vital signs, and stay with the client until an ambulance or emergency services arrive. If the client is in the early stages of insulin shock, call the supervisor to get physician orders and a nurse to come to the client's home.

Because there are many of the same symptoms in both hyperglycemic coma and insulin shock, the HCA must look at obvious differences such as skin condition, sweet breath odor, and the presence or absence of nausea and vomiting. It may be helpful to keep the symptoms of both posted in a visible place. Table 5–1 shows the differences between hyperglycemic coma and insulin shock.

Helpful Hints: The specially trained HCA should ask the nurse for signs to post at the client's home.

Table 5–1 Differences between Diabetic Coma and Insulin Shock	
Diabetic Coma (Hyperglycemia)	**InsulinShock (Hypoglycemia)**
Gradual onset	Sudden onset
Drowsiness	Nervousness
Deep, difficult breathing	Shallow breathing
Nausea	Hunger
Hot, flushed, dry skin	Moist, pale skin
Mental confusion	Mental confusion
	Vision disturbance
Loss of consciousness	Loss of consciousness
Sweet (fruity) odor on breath	

In these emergency situations, the HCA's role is careful observing and reporting, as well as accurate documentation of the incident, including who was notified, messages left, family members present, and emergency medical service professional's name.

REVIEW QUESTIONS

1. Five acute complications associated with diabetes are _____ , _____ , _____ , _____ and _____ .

2. Hunger and blurred vision are symptoms of _____ .

3. A complication occurring in response to a sudden need for insulin brought on by illness or injury is _____

4. If the client with diabetes appears to be in a ketoacidotic state, the HCA should call _____ and _____ , and should always be careful to document every detail observed.

5. In emergency situations, the HCA's role is careful observing and reporting, as well as accurate documentation of the incident, including _____ , _____ , _____ , and emergency medical service professional's name.

6. Which of the following are signs and symptoms of hyperglycemia?

   a. appetite

   b. weakness

   c. increased thirst

   d. all of the above

7. Which of these complications are not associated with hyperglycemic coma?

   a. hypertension

   b. dehydration

   c. slow heart rate (pulse)

   d. fever

8. Insulin shock is caused by.
   a. skipping a meal
   b. excessive exercise
   c. too much food
   d. nausea

9. Which is not true of foot complications?
   a. caused by poor circulation
   b. high risk of becoming infected in diabetics
   c. caused by excessive perspiration
   d. they may lead to gangrene

10. True or False? PVD increases the risk for amputations.

11. True or False? Infections in diabetic clientss may lead to ketoacidosis.

12. Unscramble the following key term from the chapter: nlusiin kscoh _____ _____

CHAPTER 6

Chronic Complications

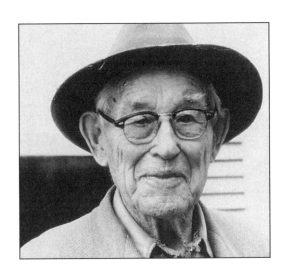

OBJECTIVES

Upon reading this chapter and completing the review questions, the home care aide should be able to:

1. Describe the focus of client care in the important area of prevention of chronic complications including eye problems, infections, injuries, and skin breakdown.

2. Define proper ways to manage stress experienced by the diabetic client and his or her family.

3. Describe the guidelines for caring for the client with diabetes when the client has another illness such as a cold or the flu.

KEY WORDS

cardiovascular disease   gangrene

chronic complication

INTRODUCTION

This chapter addresses some important complications and discusses the special care involved when the diabetic person has an

chronic complication   an illness or disorder that develops slowly over time, but may last for the client's lifetime.

illness not related to diabetes. A **chronic complication** is a disorder that develops slowly and may last for a client's whole lifetime. Some chronic complications associated with Diabetes Mellitus include the following:

- vascular problems
- eye disorders
- neuropathies
- infections
- poor skin integrity
- stress

VASCULAR PROBLEMS

Peripheral vascular disease (poor circulation or any abnormal condition affecting the blood vessels outside the heart) increases the risk for lower extremity ulcers and amputations, and for chronic heart disease (see Figure 6–1). The signs and symptoms are numbness, pain, and paleness of extremities. Changes in arteries occur in the diabetic person at an earlier age than normal.

cardiovascular disease   any abnormal condition related to the heart and its blood vessels.

Cardiovascular disease is any abnormal condition related to the heart and its blood vessels, and also occurs in persons with diabetes. In fact, persons with diabetes are twice as likely to die of heart disease than are people not affected by the disease. Hypertension is twice as common in these patients as well. The American Heart Association guidelines for all persons for the prevention of heart disease include:

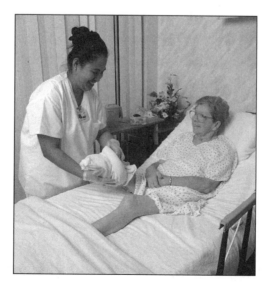

Figure 6–1   Poor circulation increases the risk for lower extremity ulcers, amputations, and chronic heart disease.

Helpful Hints: Low-cholesterol diets for diabetic patients should be chosen by the physician or dietitian to determine daily carbohydrate intake levels for the client.

- maintaining normal weight
- exercising on a regular basis
- keeping blood pressure at normal levels
- keeping cholesterol at normal levels

These guidelines, and strict adherence to them, are especially important for the diabetic client who is at a higher risk for health problems than the normal, healthy person.

EYE DISORDERS

Retinopathy (disease of the eye leading to blindness) is prevalent in clients with diabetes. More than 80 percent of clients with diabetes develop this eye disorder 15 years following the diagnosis. There is no cure for retinopathy, and prevention is of the utmost importance for clients with diabetes. Keeping the clients blood pressure within acceptable limits is important in preventing this disorder. The client should see an opthamologist or physician who specializes in diseases of the eyes at least once a year for early detection and treatment. Other vision changes common in the client with diabetes are glaucoma, cataracts, and retinitis.

Helpful Hints: Long periods of high blood sugar are especially harmful to the eyes. When blood sugar returns to normal, the symptoms often disappear. Over the years, however, damage to the eyes occurs.

NEUROPATHY

Neuropathies are disorders of the peripheral nerves (nerves other than those of the brain or spinal cord). Peripheral neuropathies often occur in clients with diabetes as a result of blood sugar and insulin imbalance, and lead to muscle weakness, atrophy, or deformities. Usually the client experiences decreased feeling in the hands and/or feet. The client should be cautioned about signs and symptoms of neuropathies. A neuropathy can affect the cardiovascular, gastrointestinal, and genitourinary systems, and may cause sexual dysfunction. The client has disturbing symptoms caused by interference with the nerve impulses. Measures to reduce discomfort include:

- avoiding temperature extremes
- keeping hands and feet warm in cold weather
- avoiding the use of hotwater bottles or heating pads that could burn desensitized areas
- avoiding trauma and injury to lower extremities
- promoting safety measures, such as supportive devices and proper footwear

Helpful Hints: The HCA should be alert for complaints of numbness or coldness in the hands and feet of the diabetic clients.

INFECTIONS

Diabetics have lowered resistance to infection because of hyperglycemia, weakened bladders, and poor circulation. When an infection occurs, it could be dangerous because infections affect the client's blood glucose levels. Infections, which affect metabolic balance, is the most common cause of diabetic ketoacidosis. With this increased potential for infection, the HCA must use careful infection control measures, such as standard precautions and frequent hand-washing techniques. The HCA should also reinforce the use of good infection control practices for the client and family. The Centers for Disease Control (CDC) recommends that diabetics have yearly influenza vaccines to reduce the risk of acute influenza.

Foot Complications

Because of poor circulation in the extremities (usually the legs and feet) of diabetic clients, there is a higher incidence of foot complications. Infection is common when cuts or abrasions occur on the feet, and if not treated promptly, can lead to gangrene and ultimately to amputation. Care should be taken regarding proper fitting of shoes, never allowing the client to walk barefoot, and never trimming the client's toenails.

The legs and feet are especially open to infection because of poor circulation. Fungal infections between toes can cause cracks and openings for bacteria to enter the body. Infections lead to **gangrene**, a decay of tissue due to obstructed or poor blood supply, and the loss of toes and in some cases the whole foot sometimes results (see Figure 6–2). The client should take care to carefully dry between toes after showering or bathing in order to prevent infections that lead to skin breakdown.

gangrene decay and death of tissue as a result of poor or no circulation to a body part.

SKIN BREAKDOWN

Breaks in the skin can lead to infections. Health care personnel should encourage clients to bathe often, check the skin for irritation, and apply lotions for skin dryness. Lotions should be free of alcohol and fragrances which may irritate sensitive skin. Patting the skin dry rather than rubbing is best, and teaching the client

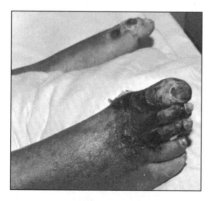

Figure 6–2 Gengrene of the toes and foot means eventual amputation.

to wear cotton underwear and socks may prevent skin break-down. If skin break downs or an ulcer occurs, the client should go to the physician immediately.

ORAL HYGIENE

Clients with diabetes must also practice careful oral hygiene to minimize gum disease and abscesses which the disease makes worse. Frequent cleaning and regular checkups, at least every six months, are most important in order to prevent these problems. Figure 6–3 shows an HCA assisting the client with oral hygiene. The biggest problem is dental plaque, a collection of bacteria, which if left on the teeth or gums, can cause tooth loss and/or gum disease.

Helpful Hints: The HCA should encourage flossing, and a medium- to soft-bristle toothbrush for oral hygiene.

STRESS

Periods of emotional stress also can cause changes in glucose levels. Having this chronic and serious disease is a stressful situation in itself. HCAs should teach clients to establish good emotional support systems, and encourage lifestyle changes that are conducive to lowering stress levels.

Red flags which indicate positive stress or psychological concerns are:

- frequent family fights over the disease
- frequent hospitalizations or medical crises
- frequent loss of days from school or work
- significant changes in blood sugar levels
- careless eating on diet
- drop in school grades or work performance

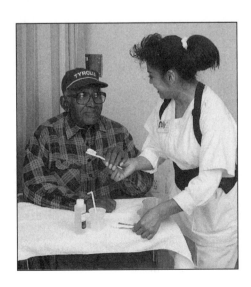

Figure 6–3 The HCA should encourage careful oral hygiene.

- major changes in mood
- major changes in relationships
- major changes in activities
- overprotective parent(s)
- overindulgent parent or significant other
- parent or significant other becomes distant after diagnosis
- age-inappropriate behavior

Stress management techniques include:
- breathing techniques
- imagery
- meditation
- biofeedback
- psychotherapy
- music therapy
- laughter; reading
- walking or exercise

OTHER ILLNESSES

When the diabetic person has a cold or the flu, blood glucose is more difficult to control. Usually, the insulin needs to be increased and closer observation undertaken to avoid complications. The following are guidelines for such prevention of complications at this important time:

- the physician should be notified if changes in medications are required
- blood glucose and urine testing should be done more often
- if nausea or vomiting occur and food intake changes, carbohydrate substitutes should be recommended by the nurse or dietitian
- HCAs should take more frequent TPRs (temperature, pulse, and respirations), and watch for signs of dehydration

When clients with diabetes have surgery, the preoperative and postoperative periods are high risk for imbalances of glucose because of abnormal food and fluid intake. The physician will order careful monitoring of blood glucose levels and intravenous infusions of insulin as required.

REVIEW QUESTIONS

1. A disorder which develops slowly and lasts a lifetime is called a _____ .
2. Poor circulation affecting blood vessels outside the heart is called _____ _____ _____ .
3. An abnormal condition related to the heart is called _____ disease.
4. The disease of the retina leading to blindness is called _____ .
5. Which of the following is not a chronic complication of diabetes?
   a. heart disease
   b. circulatory disease
   c. infections
   d. insulin shock
6. Which are measures to reduce discomfort for diabetics with neuropathy?
   a. avoid trauma to legs
   b. wear proper fitting shoes
   c. keep hands warm in the winter
   d. all of the above
7. Which is not true of foot complications?
   a. they are caused by poor circulation
   b. they can cause a high risk for infection in diabetics
   c. they are caused by excessive perspiration
   d. they may lead to gangrene
8. True or False? Peripheral vascular disease increases the risk for amputations.
9. True or False? Infections in diabetics may lead to ketoacidosis.
10. Unscramble the following key term from the chapter: eeggannr _____

Client Care

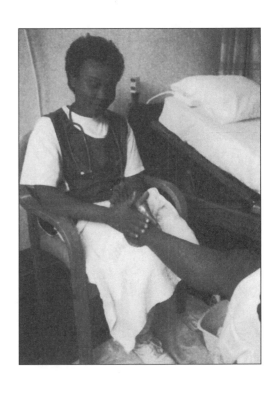

OBJECTIVES

Upon reading this chapter and completing the review questions, the home care aide should be able to:

1. Demonstrate procedures for foot care, skin care, and bowel and bladder training.
2. Collect a fresh urine specimen for testing glucose levels.
3. Assist the client with blood glucose monitoring.
4. Demonstrate the Acetest® and the Clinitest®.

KEY WORDS

Acetest®	incontinence
Clinitest®	podiatrist

INTRODUCTION

There are several client care procedures that are very important when caring for the client with diabetes. These procedures include proper foot care, proper skin care, bladder and bowel training, collecting a fresh, fractional urine specimen, blood and urine glucose testing, and urine acetone testing.

FOOT CARE

Proper foot care cannot be emphasized enough when caring for the client with diabetes. The physician and the nurse will teach the client and family proper foot care guidelines, and the specially trained HCA should reinforce these principles.

podiatrist a doctor who specializes in foot care.

Foot problems are common in clients with diabetes because of poor circulation, decreased sensation in the feet and hands, poor fitting shoes, and improper trimming of nails. Only a **podiatrist** (foot-care physician) or foot-care specialist should trim the toenails of a client with diabetes, and treat hangnails or ingrown toenails because any break in the skin of a diabetic client can lead to serious infection.

Diabetes reduces blood flow to the feet, and this creates a high risk of complications. The care should be focused on:

- self-examination of feet for skin breakdowns, ulcers, cuts, and the like
- allowing only the podiatrist or foot-care specialist to cut nails and evaluate corns and bunions
- carefully select shoes and activities
- prevention of foot injuries, such as those that occur with hot water or an electric blanket
- avoiding bare feet and tight shoes
- avoiding tight socks or stockings
- avoiding crossing the legs
- checking the inside of shoes to remove any objects

Proper foot care prevents injury and infection. Feet should be washed daily and patted dry. Vaseline® or fragrance-free, alcohol-free lotion can also be applied, but not between the toes. Properly fitted shoes should always be worn by clients with diabetes because bare feet are at too great a risk for these persons. Refer to Procedure 1 for client foot care.

CLIENT CARE PROCEDURE

1   Giving Foot and Toenail Care

NOTE: Check with the nurse and the nursing care plan to determine if this procedure is permitted for the patient, or if it is to be modified because of the patient's condition. Older patients are more comfortable during this procedure if you squat so they do not have to extend their legs.

1. Carry out each beginning procedure action.
2. Remember to wash your hands, identify the patient, and provide privacy.

1   Giving Foot and Toenail Care

3. Assemble equipment needed:
   - wash basin
   - soap
   - bath mat
   - lotion
   - disposable bed protector
   - bath towel/washcloth
   - orangewood stick
4. If permitted, assist patient out of bed and into a chair.
5. Place bath mat on floor in front of patient.
6. Fill basin with warm water (105ºF). Place basin on bath mat.
7. Remove slippers and allow patient to place feet in water (Figure 7–1A). Cover with bath towel to help retain heat (Figure 7–1B).

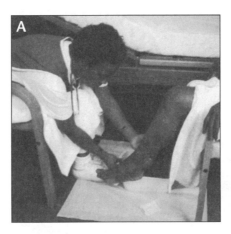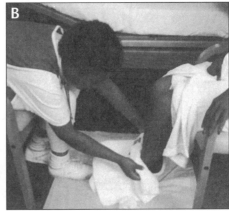

Figure 7–1 (A) Soak client's feet in warm water. (B) Cover feet and basin with towel to retain warmth.

8. Soak feet approximately 20 minutes.
   - add warm water as necessary
   - lift feet from water while warm water is being added (Figure 7–1C).
9. At end of soak period:
   - wash feet with soap
   - use washcloth to gently scrub roughened areas
   - rinse and dry (Figure 7–1D).
   - note any abnormalities such as corns or callouses
10. Remove basin and cover feet with towel.
11. Use the orangewood stick to gently clean toenails (Figure 7–1E). If nails are long and need to be cut, report this to the nurse. *Do not* undertake this task yourself.
12. Dry feet.

1   Giving Foot and Toenail Care

13. Pour lotion into the palms of your hands, and hold hands together to warm lotion. Apply to patient's feet (Figure 7–1F). *Do not* apply lotion between the toes.

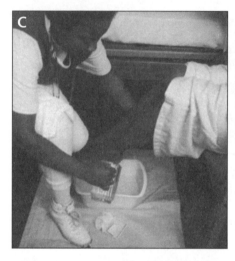
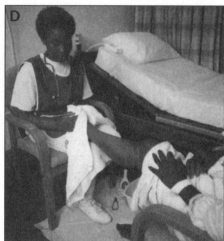

Figure 7–1(continued) (C) Lift feet while warm water is being added. (D) Dry feet gently, especially between toes, and inspect for any abnormalities.

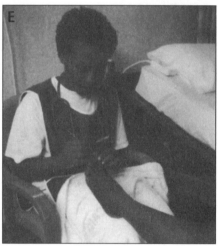
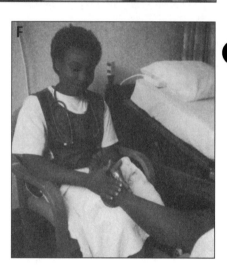

Figure 7–1 (continued) (E) Clean toenails carefully with an orangewood stick. (F) Gently apply lotion to the patient's feet.

14. Assist patient with slippers and to return to bed unless ambulatory.

15. Carry out each procedure completion action. Remember to wash your hands, report completion of task, and document date, time, foot and toenail care, and patient reaction.

SKIN CARE

Helpful Hints: Foot care and inspection of the feet for injury and infection by the HCA should be done on every client visit.

Caring for the skin is important for the client with diabetes because this client has poor circulation. Skin breakdown, once it occurs, is extremely difficult to heal. Changes occur in the nerve endings, and the client's sense of hot or cold may be impaired. Burns can occur more easily in the client with diabetes.

incontinence   inability of a person to control bowel or bladder function.

Skin care is given to clients with diabetes to prevent breakdown of the skin which causes pressure sores. When there is pressure, shearing, or friction on the skin, breakdown occurs. Contributing factors may include lack of cleanliness, moisture (such as perspiration or urine), **incontinence**, poor nutrition, or soap left on the skin. The skin breaks down in four stages:

Stage I: Redness lasting longer than 30 minutes after pressure is removed; the area my be warm to touch (Figure 7–2).

Stage II: The skin is reddened, and has a blister or broken area on the skin surface (Figure 7–3).

Stage III: Layers of the skin have been destroyed, and may or may not include infection (Figure 7–4).

Stage IV: Skin is gone, and the ulcer is deep into muscle and bone (Figure 7–5).

Seven ways to prevent skin breakdown are:

1.   Remove pressure from bony areas.

2.   Massage the skin surrounding the area.

3.   Keep skin clean and dry.

4.   Reposition the client frequently.

5.   Remove urine and feces from the skin promptly.

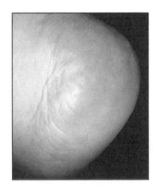

Figure 7–2   Stage I: The first sign of a pressure ulcer is redness lasting longer than 30 minutes after pressure is removed. The area may also be warm to the touch. (Courtesy: Emory University Hospital, Atlanta, Georgia.)

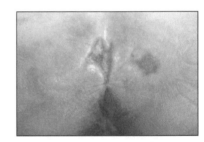

Figure 7–3   Stage II: The skin is reddened and has a blister or broken area on the surface. (Courtesy: Emory University Hospital, Atlanta, Georgia.)

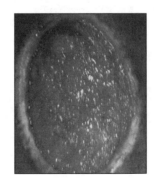

Figure 7–4   Stage III: Layers of the skin have been destroyed and may include infection. (Courtesy: Emory University Hospital, Atlanta, Georgia.)

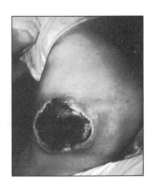

Figure 7–5   Stage IV: Skin is gone, and the ulcer is deep into the muscle and bone. (Courtesy: Emory University Hospital, Atlanta, Georgia.)

6. Pat skin dry instead of rubbing.

7. Give back massages.

The client's skin should be observed regularly and accurately, especially at pressure points. Figure 7–6 shows the most common sites for pressure sores. The HCA should report any changes in the skin, such as redness, heat, tenderness, or blisters immediately. Incontinent clients should be checked for dryness frequently (every one to two hours). Depends™ and other disposable briefs should be changed frequently. Preventative devices can be sheepskin heel and elbow protectors and bed cradles. Figure 7–7 shows various preventative devices used to lower the chances of skin breakdown.

HCAs should follow the guidelines set down by their agencies or facilities for special skin care programs. Cleanliness is the main objective, along with careful observation. The HCA and/or the family can apply special creams and ointments as directed by the nurse or supervisor if there are no signs of infections or open wounds on the area, and stimulate circulation in the back, buttocks, and bony areas through massage. Refer to Procedure 2 for special skin care and pressure sores.

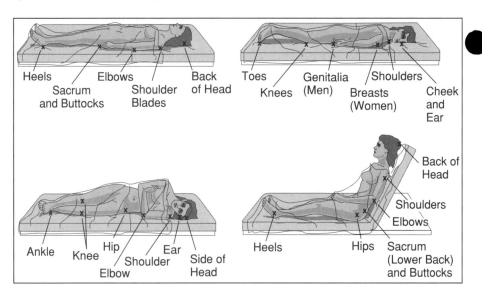

Figure 7–6 The most common sites for pressure sores.

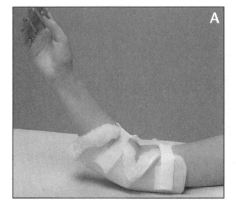 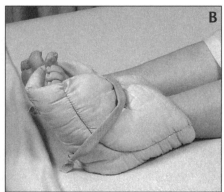

Figure 7–7 (A) Elbow pads reduce skin irritation. (Courtesy: J. T. Posey Company, Arcadia, California.) (B) Foot pads prevent friction and reduce the chance of infection.

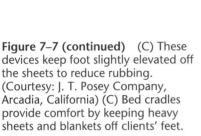

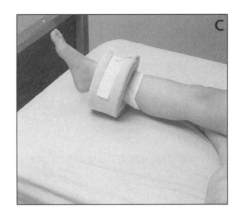

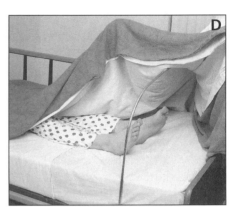

Figure 7–7 (continued) (C) These devices keep foot slightly elevated off the sheets to reduce rubbing. (Courtesy: J. T. Posey Company, Arcadia, California) (C) Bed cradles provide comfort by keeping heavy sheets and blankets off clients' feet.

CLIENT CARE PROCEDURE

2   Special Skin Care and Pressure Sores

PURPOSE

- To prevent skin breakdown resulting from pressure and skin irritations
- To use preventive devices
- To prevent friction resulting when skin is in contact with skin or linen.

   NOTE: Certain clients are at risk for the development of pressure sores, such as clients who are bedridden, obese, emaciated, diabetic, paralyzed, and malnourished. A home health aide's role is mainly to prevent pressure sore development. Once a pressure sore has developed, the nurse will have to come to the client's home to treat the open area.

ASSISTIVE DEVICES TO PREVENT PRESSURE SORES

1. Air mattress—This is a mattress filled with air, and works by continuously changing the pressure areas on the client's back. One can improvise an air mattress designed for camping instead of buying a medical air mattress.

2. Egg crate mattress—This is a mattress made of foam rubber that is molded like an egg crate. They are inexpensive but effective in reducing pressure on the skin. One also can be purchased for the seat of a chair for the client to sit on during the day.

3. Water mattress—This is similar to a regular water mattress used in homes. This mattress is effective in reducing pressure on the skin, but causes problems when transferring clients into and out of bed.

4. Gel foam cushion—This is a special cushion filled with a special solution of gel. This style of cushion is effective in the prevention of pressure sores for a client who sits in a wheelchair for long periods of time.

5. Sheepskin or lamb's wool pads, or elbow or heel pads—Lamb's wool pads prevent pressure sores by acting as a barrier between the client's skin and the sheets.

6. Bed cradle—This is a device to keep linens off the client's legs and feet. In the home care setting, a client can substitute a box or other device to keep linens off legs and feet.

CLIENT CARE PROCEDURE, *continued*

2   Special Skin Care and Pressure Sores

SPECIAL CARE TO PREVENT PRESSURE SORES

1. Change client's position at least every two hours to reduce pressure on any one area.
2. As quickly as possible, remove feces, urine, or moisture of any kind that might be irritating to the skin.
3. Encourage clients who sit in chairs or wheelchairs to raise themselves or change position every 15 minutes to relieve pressure.
4. Encourage clients to eat a high-protein diet, if allowed, and to drink adequate fluids.
5. Keep bed linens clean, dry, and wrinkle-free.
6. When bathing clients, use soap sparingly because soap dries the skin. Keep the client's skin well lubricated.
7. Watch for skin irritation when applying braces and splints.
8. At the first sign of a reddened area, gently massage area around the spot. Report your observations to the nurse or supervisor.

Helpful Hints: Skin care should be done on every visit for elderly, diabetic clients.

In addition, the bedbound client should be repositioned every two hours to prevent skin breakdown. The more active client should be encouraged to ambulate as much as is safely possible.

The client with diabetes should bathe frequently and gently pat the skin dry. HCAs should carefully check the temperature of water for bathing and showering of clients so the client is not burned. The HCA should instruct the client to always check the temperature of the bath or shower before entering in order to prevent burns. Hot water heaters should not be set above 101ºF. Lotions and creams are beneficial to prevent dry skin areas which may quickly break down. The HCA should read the labels of the lotions used by the client to ensure they are free of fragrances and alcohol. Any open or reddened areas on the client's skin should be reported to the supervisor, and the physician notified quickly so that proper action can be taken to prevent skin breakdown. Blisters, scratches, and sores can be very dangerous, and may heal poorly. Skin should be carefully observed during baths and dressing.

BOWEL AND BLADDER TRAINING

Bowel and bladder training is an important process for clients with elimination dysfunction and incontinence. Incontinence is the inability to control urination or the bowels. Some clients with diabetes have lost all or part of their control, and in some cases, the physician and the nurse may determine that bowel or bladder rehabilitation training may be useful in regaining some or all of this function. Sometimes, incontinence can be prevented by offering the bedpad or urinal to the client on a regular schedule

For bowel training, the physician may order suppositories which stimulate the rectum for a bowel movement. The HCA may be asked to assist the client in inserting the suppository. When doing so, the HCA should observe the client's ability to control his or her bowels, particularly in terms of how long the bowel movement can be retained. Occasionally, enemas are ordered as part of bowel training. The HCA should check first with the supervisor to determine the agency's policy and procedure for giving or assisting with enemas. Commercially prepared enemas are usually approved for HCA use, but the HCA should review the Department of Health regulations in his or her state to ensure this procedure is approved. Oil-retention enemas are also commercially prepared. The client should retain the oil for as long as possible in bed in a quiet position. These enemas are especially useful for constipation as a result of dehydration.

Some areas to focus on in bowel training are:

- observing the bowel pattern by keeping a record of the time and character of each bowel movement
- having the nurse check for fecal impactions
- observing for signs of constipation or diarrhea
- reporting any abdominal or rectal discomfort
- establishing regularity by offering the bedpan or beside commode at regular times
- assisting the client with bowel aides such as suppositories or laxatives as prescribed by the physician
- offering a comfortable and private environment for the client to move his or her bowels
- offering a warm drink to stimulate the bowel movement if the client is unsuccessful

Adequate fluid intake is an important part of bowel training to prevent constipation. Sometimes a diet with increased fiber may be ordered by the physician. Bowel training can take up to eight weeks, and consistent support from the caregiver is essential. Refer to Procedure 3 for bowel training.

Helpful Hints: Warming oil enemas in water before giving them to the client increases their effectiveness.

Helpful Hints: Clients who perspire excessively in warm weather may become dehydrated easily. This leads to constipation.

CLIENT CARE PROCEDURE

3 **Training and Retraining Bowels**

PURPOSE

- To train a client to be continent of bowel movement
- To regulate a client to have regular bowel movement.

3   Training and Retraining Bowels

NOTE: Constipation can result from illness, poor eating habits, drug therapy, and lack of exercise. Constipation causes the client added discomfort when it occurs in addition to other physical problems. An individualized bowel program is designed by the health care team for each client. For example, one client may regulate his or her bowels by adding prune juice to the diet twice a day, whereas another client may have to drink daily prune juice and take a daily laxative and stool softener as well.

Older clients can become overly "bowel conscious," and have a misconception of what normal elimination should be. The frequency of bowel movements may range from three times a day for one person to only once every two or three days for another. Therefore, the term constipation should not be used to describe a missed movement or two, but only the unusual retention of fecal matter along with infrequent or difficult passage of stony, hard stool.

Among the elderly, constipation is very often encountered. If a client is unable to exercise and move about regularly, bowel action becomes sluggish. In addition, medications, especially painkillers, can cause constipation. If a client has hemorrhoids, there may be a fear of pain and the client avoids trying to have a bowel movement. If a client does not have a bowel movement for a few days, he or she may develop an impaction. An impaction is a large amount of hard stool in the lower colon or rectum. This is a very painful condition. If a client does develop an impaction, the nurse will have to remove it manually.

PROCEDURE

1. Health care team assesses prior habits of client. If the client has always had a bowel movement early in the morning, this is important to know in planning the client's retraining program.

2. A plan is designed and implemented. Important elements of the plan are:
   - high intake of fiber foods
   - adequate intake of liquids
   - regular exercise
   - toileting of client at regular intervals
   - praise by aide at slightest progress of client
   - less reliance on laxatives and enemas
   - privacy for client during bowel movements

3. Follow bowel retraining program developed by the health care team. If plan appears to be working, note success of program. If plan does not work, report to the nurse or supervisor. It is also important to give some suggestions to the health care team of possible solutions for retraining the client.

Bladder training is most often ordered for clients who have problems with retention of urine or incontinence. Retraining the bladder takes from six to eight weeks and emotional support is a big factor. Figure 7–8 shows an example of a bladder retraining assessment. All members of the health care team, the client, and the family need to know what the training program is and how to play a role. The same is true for bowel training as well as bladder training. The client and family's participation and cooperation are vital to the success of the program.

Some of the areas to focus on in bladder retraining are:

- Encouraging fluids in the daytime hours and restricting them at night.

- When offering the bedpan or commode, positioning is important. The height of the seat and handrails can offer comfort for the client. Men find it easier to urinate in a standing position.

- Additional stimuli may encourage voiding (urinating) such as offering a glass of water, pouring warm water over the perineum, running water in the sink, bearing down to empty the bladder (unless contraindicated by the physician), and placing the patient's hand in warm water.

- Cleaning the skin on the incontinent client on a regular basis.

- Offering to assist the client to urinate on a regular schedule (every three to four hours).

- Keeping a careful report of the time and amount of urination on the record and on the intake and output sheets.

Refer to Procedure 4 for retraining the bladder.

CLIENT CARE PROCEDURE

4   Retraining the Bladder

PURPOSE

- To regain bladder control

PROCEDURE

A home health aide should keep a record of how often and how much the client voids throughout the day and night for a few days. Once the client's voiding pattern is known, the nurse or supervisor can analyze the client's voiding record and formulate a schedule for the aide to follow. The schedule developed by the nurse will include regularly scheduled times for the aide to have the client drink a measured amount of fluid. After the client had drunk the liquid, the aide notes the time. Thirty minutes later the aide should toilet the client. The aide will need to encourage the client to void each time he or she is positioned on the commode or toilet. It is helpful at times to run water from the faucet to give the client an urge to void. Other methods of encour-

BLADDER RETRAINING ASSESSMENT
(Reference tags: F315, F316)

CURRENT CLIENT STATUS

DIAGNOSIS_____ RESIDENT'S AGE_____

RECENT SURGERY? ☐ Yes ☐ No If Yes, date_____/_____/_____ and type_____

CURRENT MEDICATIONS (i.e., Diuretics, Psychotropics, etc.)_____

_____

_____

Mental Status and Ability to Communicate	Mobility Status	Vision Status	Right	Left
☐ Alert	☐ Independent	Adequate	☐	☐
☐ Aphasic	☐ Transfer/standing ability	Adequate w/aid	☐	☐
☐ Oriented x_____	☐ Wheelchair bound	Poor	☐	☐
☐ Disoriented	☐ Bed rest	Blind	☐	☐
☐ Depressed	☐ Contractures	**Hearing Status**	**Right**	**Left**
☐ Cooperative	☐ Other_____			
☐ Uncooperative	_____	Adequate	☐	☐
☐ Slow comprehension	_____	Adequate w/aid	☐	☐
☐ Other_____	_____	Poor	☐	☐
		Deaf	☐	☐

BLADDER ASSESSMENT

1. **LENGTH OF INCONTINENCE:** _____ Days _____ Months _____ Years

2. **REASON FOR INCONTINENCE (if known):** _____

   CATHETER: ☐ Yes ☐ No If Yes, specify type and size _____

   Date inserted _____/_____/_____ Reason for catheter _____

3. **USUAL VOIDING PATTERN:** Frequency_____ Amt./voiding_____ cc: /24 hrs._____ cc

   Pattern: ☐ Upon arising ☐ After meals ☐ No apparent pattern ☐ Night time only

   ☐ Other (specify)_____

4. **SYMPTOMS:** (Check all that apply)
   - ☐ Voids often in small amounts ☐ Difficulty stopping stream ☐ Urgency
   - ☐ Fills bladder/voids large amount ☐ Dribbles constantly ☐ Burning/Pain
   - ☐ Unable to void ☐ Dribbles after voiding ☐ Edema
   - ☐ Difficulty starting stream ☐ Dribbles while coughing ☐ Other (specify)_____

5. **HISTORY OF:** ☐ Urinary Disorders ☐ Bladder Disorders ☐ Kidney Disease ☐ Prostate Problems
   ☐ Neurological Disorders ☐ Fecal Impactions ☐ Other (specify)_____

6. **RELIEF AFTER VOIDING:** ☐ Complete ☐ Continued desire to void

7. **BLADDER DISTENDED:** ☐ Yes ☐ No **EMPTIED BY EXTERNAL STIMULI:** ☐ Yes ☐ No

   If Yes, Check: ☐ Kegel Exercises ☐ Warm water over perineum

   ☐ Other (specify)_____

8. **RESIDUAL URINE:** ☐ Yes ☐ No If Yes, Amount: _____ cc

9. **PERCEPTION OF NEED TO VOID:** ☐ Present ☐ Diminished ☐ Absent

10. **WELL HYDRATED:** ☐ Yes ☐ No **AVERAGE FLUID INTAKE (24 HRS)** _____ cc

    AVERAGE FLUID OUTPUT (24 HRS) _____ cc

    Fluids Preferred _____

NAME—Last	First	Middle	Attending Physician	Chart No.

BLADDER RETRAINING ASSESSMENT
☐ Continued on Reverse

Figure 7–8 Bladder retraining assessment sheet *(continues)*

Comp.#1983 Page 2, Film 1, One Color, Backer for HH

EVALUATION FOR BLADDER RETRAINING POTENTIAL

☐ **ABLE TO PARTICIPATE IN RETRAINING**   EVALUATION PERIOD: _____ TO _____

PLAN: _____

_____

PROVIDE FLUIDS:	FLUIDS SHOULD BE SPACED AS FOLLOWS:					
_____ cc every 24 Hrs	☐7AM	☐11	☐3PM	☐7	☐11PM	☐3
_____ cc 7-3 shift	☐8	☐12N	☐4	☐8	☐12MN	☐4
_____ cc 3-11 shift	☐9	☐1PM	☐5	☐9	☐1AM	☐5
_____ cc 11-7 shift	☐10	☐2	☐6	☐10	☐2	☐6

OFFER NO FLUIDS AFTER _____ PM   **TOILET FOR VOIDING EVERY** ___ Hrs (Day and Evening) ___ Hrs (Night)
(Except as needed for medications)
RECORD RESULTS ON BLADDER RETRAINING RECORD.

☐ **UNABLE TO PARTICIPATE IN RETRAINING**

REASON: _____

_____

REEVALUATION DATE: _____

COMPLETED BY: _____   ___ / ___ / ___
                          Signature/Title   Date

BLADDER RETRAINING PROGRESS NOTES OR REEVALUATION NOTES

DATE	TIME	NOTES - ALL ENTRIES MUST BE SIGNED WITH NAME AND TITLE

NAME—Last	First	Middle	Attending Physician	Chart No.

BLADDER RETRAINING NOTES

Figure 7-8 *continued*

4   Retraining the Bladder

aging the client to void are to have the client apply light pressure to the bladder area to stimulate the urge to empty the bladder, or have the client lean forward on the toilet to stimulate emptying the bladder. Remember that the client needs to be toileted at regular intervals to prevent accidents. The client also needs consistent positive reinforcement to remain dry. At first, it may be necessary to take the client to the bathroom every two hours; intervals may be lengthened as control is gained. A common cause of incontinence is delay in getting the client to the bathroom. It is of utmost importance to take the client to the bathroom on a regular time schedule. The plan will also call for the aide to maintain the client's fluid intake at about 2500 cc/day. The aide should encourage the client to wear regular underwear to enhance the client's self-esteem, and to help the client from reverting back to the previous habit of incontinence.

COLLECTING A FRESH, FRACTIONAL URINE SPECIMEN

Because the client with diabetes may spill glucose into the urine when hyperglycemic, the HCA may be asked to collect a fresh urine specimen for testing. The term "fresh urine" refers to urine recently collected from the bladder. Therefore, the first urine voided in the morning must not be used as a fresh specimen. Rather, it should be discarded and a fresh one obtained. Urine that has accumulated overnight will not reflect the level of glucose in the urine at the time of the test. This fresh specimen can usually be taken from the first voiding after the morning void, (usually 30 minutes later because only a small amount is required). Refer to Procedure 5 for collecting a fresh, fractional urine specimen.

5   Collecting a Fresh, Fractional Urine Specimen

1. Carry out each beginning procedure action.
2. Remember to wash your hands, identify the patient, and provide privacy.
3. Assemble equipment needed:
   - two specimen containers
   - urinal or bedpan
   - testing materials if urine testing is to be performed (Ketostix®)
   - small plastic bag for used toilet tissue
   - disposable gloves

5 Collecting a Fresh, Fractional Urine Specimen

4. About one hour before testing is to be done, wash your hands and take equipment to bedside: take an initial sample at this time, and a smaller sample in one hour or less.

5. Screen unit and offer the bedpan or urinal (the patient may be assisted to the commode, if permitted).

6. Put on disposable gloves.

7. Encourage patient to empty bladder.

8. Do not permit tissue to be placed in receptacle. Place in plastic bag and discard.

9. Take receptacle to bathroom or utility room.

10. Pour sample into one specimen container. Test this sample in case patient fails to void a second time.

11. Make a note of the test result, but do not record it officially.

12. Clean equipment according to facility policy and return to the proper area. Measure and record urine if patient is on I & O.

13. Remove and dispose of gloves according to facility policy.

14. Wash your hands.

15. Offer water for the patient to wash his or her hands.

16. If permitted, encourage patient to drink water. Be sure to record intake on I & O sheet.

17. Tell patient when you will return for the second sample. Return to the patient's unit at the proper time.

18. Wash you hands and identify the patient. Explain to the client what you plan to do, and how he or she can help.

19. Repeat Steps 5–15.

20. Carry out each procedure completion action. Remember to wash your hands, report completion of task, and document time, fractional urine specimen to laboratory, and patient reaction.

TESTING URINE AND BLOOD SUGAR LEVELS

The HCA may assist in testing urine and blood sugar levels of the client at various times throughout the day. The physician will instruct the client regarding how often their body sugar levels need to be tested. The HCA may be asked to collect the urine for testing (see Procedure 5). The nurse will teach the newly diagnosed diabetic client to do his or her own blood glucose testing. The most common types of urine glucose testing are the Clinitest® and the Acetest®.

Clinitest® which is a simple urine test for glucose levels, is less accurate than blood glucose monitoring

Clinitest®

A **Clinitest®** is done to test the urine for the presence of glucose. A chemical called a reagent is combined with urine and water. A color change occurs, depending on the amount of sugar in the urine. The test may be done in the home by the family, the HCA, or the client. Most Clinitests® are done with Clinitest® tablets, Testape,® or Clinistix® strips. The results determine changes in insulin dosage or diet, so accuracy is important. The urine is usually tested four times a day; one-half hour before meals and at bedtime in unstable diabetics.

Acetest®

The urine may also be tested for acetone or ketone bodies when rapid breakdown of fat occurs. If there is a lack of insulin, fat is used for energy. Keto-Diastix® are used (similar to the Clinitest® strips) in which a change in color on the reagent substance indicates the acetone level. Refer to Procedure 6 for testing the urine for acetone. Instructions are included in the manufacturer's packages for Clinitest® and Acetest®. If the client is doing his or her own urine testing, a daily log should be kept with the testing equipment in the bathroom. The nurse will teach the client and family how to perform these tests. The specially trained HCA should caution the client not to touch the test tube or tablets during the test because the chemical could burn the skin.

Acetest® is a simple urine test done to test for ketone bodies.

6 Testing Urine for Acetone: Ketostix® Strip Test

NOTE: If the results of the blood glucose tests are above normal, the nurse may request the urine be tested for acetone.

1. Carry out each beginning procedure action.
2. Wash your hands, identify the patient, and provide privacy.
3. Assemble equipment needed:
   - disposable gloves
   - Ketostix® reagent strips
   - sample of freshly voided urine in container
4. Put on disposable gloves.
5. Remove one test strip from bottle and recap.
6. Dip one end of the test strip (the end with the reagent area) into the urine (Figure 7–9a).
7. Remove the strip and hold it horizontally.
8. Exactly fifteen seconds later, compare the strip with the color chart on the bottle label (Figure 7–9B). Match it as closely as possible to one of the colors on the chart. Do not touch wet strip to bottle label.
9. Dispose of strip and urine specimen unless orders have been given to save it.
10. Remove and properly dispose of gloves according to facility policy.

6   Testing Urine for Acetone: Ketostix® Strip Test

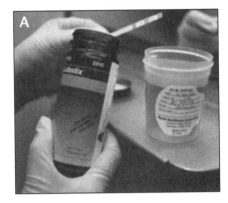
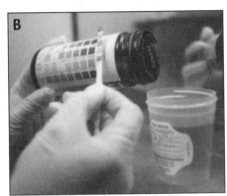

Figure 7–9   (A) Remove a test strip from bottle. Recap. Dip strip into fresh urine sample. Do not touch wet strip to label of bottle. (B) Compare strip with color chart on bottle to determine results of the urine test.

11. Carry out each procedure completion action. Remember to wash your hands, report completion of task, document time, results of urine tested for acetone using Ketostix® strip, and patient reaction.

DISPOSAL OF SHARPS

Sharps are needles, blades, disposable razors, or any instrument that can puncture the skin. The HCA who cares for a client with diabetes will probably be responsible for the disposal of numerous sharps on a daily basis. Needles should be disposed of in a puncture-resistant, leakproof container that is labeled or color coded. These containers are provided by the HCA's agency. Needles should *never* be recapped before disposal.

REVIEW QUESTION

1. A foot-care physician is called a _____ .
2. The inability to control urination or bowels is _____ .
3. Bowel training may take up to _____ weeks.
4. Two common types of urine glucose testing are the _____ and the _____ .
5. Which of the following is not considered part of skin care?
   a. applying lotion
   b. exercising the legs
   c. observation during bathing
   d. checking temperature of bath water

6. Bowel training includes:
   a. observing bowel pattern
   b. establishing regular bowel movement times
   c. adequate fluid intake
   d. all of the above
7. True or False? The client and family's participation and cooperation are important to the success of bladder training.
8. True or False? Successful voiding may be related to the position and comfort of the client.
9. True or False? Only female clients respond to additional stimuli when encouraging voiding.
10. Unscramble the following key term from the chapter: noteiniccnen _____

Client and Family Education and Support

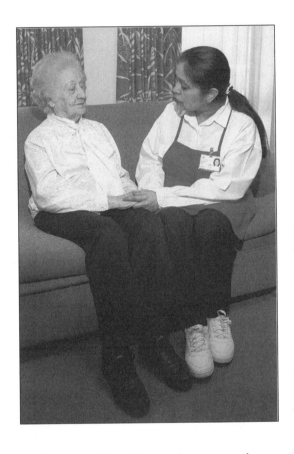

OBJECTIVES

Upon reading this chapter and completing the review questions, the home care aide should be able to:

1. Be familiar with those areas commonly included in education of the diabetic client including the disease process, the diet, complications, and exercise.

2. Understand the HCA's role in education and support.

3. Be familiar with social support that is available for the client and family.

KEY WORDS

aerobic exercise

complex carbohydrates

simple carbohydrates

Somogyi effect

INTRODUCTION

The skilled nurse will determine the client's education plan and will have printed materials that the HCA will find in the client's home. Client and family education is a skilled nursing function, but the HCA should be familiar with the content of the education plan in order to answer questions and observe the client for his or her level of understanding and utilization of the information. Many times, the skilled nurse relies on the HCA to communicate the effectiveness of the client education plan. The following are the important client education areas that should be included in every plan. The nurse first determines the client and the family's level of knowledge prior to beginning the course. Health caregivers are first educated themselves, before the client and family's education begins. Areas included in the client and family's education plan are the disease process, diet, complications, exercise, and social support.

THE DISEASE PROCESS

The disease process of Diabetes Mellitus includes an understanding of the body and how it is affected by the disease. It also includes a basic knowledge of diabetes, its signs and symptoms, how it progresses, how it affects all the body systems, knowledge about the pancreas and insulin production, and how and why unstable conditions occur. The education begins with a general overview of anatomy and physiology of the endocrine system, specifically hormones and insulin secretion. From there, it progresses to the individual types of diabetes, and the present and expected progression of the disease. A definition of diabetes and its specific types, with special emphasis on the type with which the client has been diagnosed, should be included. For a review of these factors, refer to Chapters 1 and 2.

DIET

Dietitians and nutritional counselors are trained and educated to be experts in diabetic diet management. The HCA, however, must also be knowledgeable on this subject, because clients will frequently rely on them to answer simple questions about their diets.

This includes not only understanding what diet is ordered and why, but also how to shop for and prepare the correct foods. The physician and dietitian are not in the home where the situation can be closely watched. Most home care clients rely on the home health team for education. In complicated dietary problems, a dietitian will go to the home for a visit. Therefore, the specially trained HCA should learn to help answer the following five questions:

1. When should the client eat?
2. What should the client eat?
3. How should the food be prepared?

Helpful Hints: HCAs and the family should include foods that the client likes when planning the menus for the week.

4. How should the food be purchased?

5. What happens when the client becomes ill?

The client's diet management program will include teaching from the doctor or nurse concerning the disease and the diet regimen. An important factor is to convince the clients that some control over this disease is in their hands, particularly in terms of managing their diet and nutrition. Table 8–1 shows the nutritional terms and their definitions.

Table 8–1 Nutritional Terms		
Word	**Definition**	**Examples**
Carbohydrates	Sugars or starches which are made up of carbon, hydrogen, and oxygen, and deliver quick energy to the body.	Found in grains, potatoes, corn, fruits, and sweets
Proteins	Compounds composed of amino acids needed for growth and tissue repair.	Found in meats, fish, milk, eggs, nuts, dried beans
Fats	Oily substances made up of glycerin and fatty acids, which provide stored energy to the body, and protect vital organs.	Present in meats, butter, milk, peanuts
Minerals	Inorganic elements essential in tissue-building and in regulation of body fluids.	Iron, calcium, sodium, and zinc
Vitamins	Organic substances vital to certain metabolic functions and needed to prevent deficiency disease. Vitamins are needed only in small amounts but must be obtained from food sources since they are not produced in the body.	Vitamins A, C, B_{12}
Water	A tasteless, odorless liquid compound of hydrogen and oxygen necessary in the digestive process and to regulate body processes.	
Calorie	A measure of heat produced by the body when using a specific portion of food.	
Metabolism	Sum total of processes needed for the breakdown of food and absorption of nutrients.	

The nutritionist (or dietitian) and the physician will prescribe a calculated American Diabetes Association (ADA) diet based on sound dietary principle and restriction. These include:

- the effect of food on insulin fluctuations and blood glucose levels
- the importance of maintenance of optimal body weight
- the importance of eating at regular times
- the signs and symptoms of insulin shock and hyperglycemia, and the dietary impact on each

- the effect of physical and/or emotional stress on blood sugar and any dietary implication.

There are four basic food groups that the dietitian uses to establish the client's diet (Figure 8–1). These include:

1. Dairy
2. Meats
3. Grains
4. Fruits and vegetables

Ensuring that the client has a proper supply of vitamins each day is important. Table 8–2 shows the vitamins to be included in the client's daily diet, their sources, and their functions.

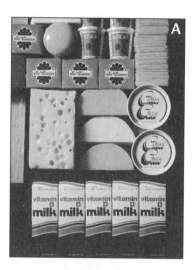
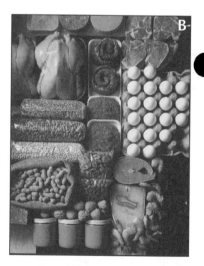
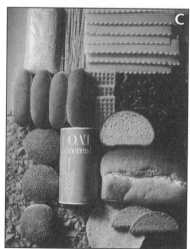
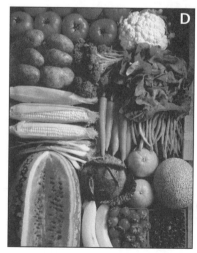

Figure 8–1   (A) The dairy group contains milk and foods that come from milk such as cheese and yogurt. (B) The meat group contains poultry, fish, dry beans, eggs, and nuts. (C) The grain group contains all kinds of breads, rice, cereals, and pasta. (D) The fruit and vegetable group contains all plants that are not in the grain group. (From How to Eat for Good Health, Courtesy National Dairy Council®).

Table 8–2 Vitamins and Their Sources		
Vitamins	**Best Sources**	**Functions**
Fat-Soluble Vitamins		
Vitamin A	Vegetables (dark green and deep yellow): Fish liver oils Liver Egg yolk Fruits (yellow)	Essential for: Growth Health of eyes Stucture and functioning of the cells of the skin and mucuous membranes
Vitamin D	Sunshine Fish liver oil Milk (irradiated) Egg yolk Liver	Essential for: Growth Regulating calcium and phosphorus metabolism Building and maintaining normal bones and teeth
Vitamin E	Wheat germ/wheat germ oils Vegetable oils Margarine Legumes Nuts Dark green, leafy vegetables	Not conclusively defined in humans; may affect the red blood cells Recommended for middle-aged women as it helps in the metabolism of calcium
Vitamin K	Spinach Kale Cabbage Cauliflower Pork liver	Essential for: Normal clotting of blood
Water-Soluble Vitamins		
Vitamin C (Ascorbic acid)	Citrus fruits, pineapple Melons and berries Tomatoes Broccoli Green peppers	Essential for: Maintaining strength of blood vessels Health of teeth and gums Aids in wound healing
Thiamine (B_1)	Wheat germ Lean pork Yeast Legumes Whole grain and enriched cereal products Liver, other organ meats	Essential for: Carbohydrate metabolism Healthy appetite Functioning of nerves
Riboflavin	Milk, cheese Enriched breads and cereals Yeast Green, leafy vegetables Eggs Liver, kidney, heart	Essential for: Health of skin, eyes, and mouth Carbohydrate, fat, and protein metabolism
Niacin (Nicotinic acid)	Meats (especially organ meats) Poultry and fish Yeast Enriched breads and cereals Peanuts	Essential for: Prevention of pellagra Carbohydrate, fat, and protein metabolism
Vitamin B_6 (Pyridoxine)	Wheat germ Liver and kidney Meats Whole grain cereals Soybeans and peanuts	Essential for: Metabolism of proteins

Continues

Table 8–2	Continued	
Vitamins	**Best Sources**	**Functions**
Pantothenic Acid	Heart, liver, kidney Eggs Peanuts Whole grain cereals	Aids various steps in metabolism
Biotin	Organ meats Yeast Mushrooms Peanuts	Aids various steps in metabolism
Vitamin B$_{12}$ (Cobalamin)	Liver, kidney Muscle meats Milk, cheese Eggs	Essential for: Metabolism Healthy red blood cells Treatment of pernicious anemia
Folacin (Folic acid)	Dark green, leafy vegetables LIver, kidney Yeast	Essential for: The blood-forming system Metabolism

For clients who take insulin (oral or injectable) as well as those who are non-insulin dependent, the timing of meals is critical. The following are guidelines to follow:

- For clients who take insulin, the type of insulin in terms of onset of action should be considered in conjunction with the client's preferred mealtime plan. Regular and consistent mealtimes are essential to the balance of insulin and glucose levels.
- Skipping meals can be very dangerous for these clients. A time delay of not more than 30 minutes is appropriate. These clients should carry a source of fast-acting carbohydrate.

The following food or food supplements contain 10 and 15 grams of rapid-acting carbohydrates, which will stabilize a client, usually within 15 minutes, who has had a mild hypoglycemic reaction:

- 3 glucose tablets
- 4 ounces orange juice
- 6 ounces regular soda
- 6 to 8 ounces 2 percent fat or skim milk
- 6 to 8 lifesavers
- 3 graham crackers
- 6 jelly beans
- 2 tablespoons of raisins
- 1 small (2-ounce) tube of cake icing

There are also over-the-counter glucose products sold as fast-acting products for diabetics to use for mild reactions. HCAs may assist the client to use them.

● **Somogyi effect** is the sudden rise in blood sugar levels early in the morning.

●

● • **Somogyi effect** may occur in the morning, and is the result of nighttime hyperglycemia in which the counterregulatory hormones overcorrect for hypoglycemia during the night. Also called "dawn phenomenon," the blood sugar tends to rise in the early morning (4 to 8 A.M.) because of an insulin clearance, insulin sensitivity, and/or counterregulatory hormones. It is important that these clients monitor blood glucose levels and also counseled on appropriate bedtime snacks.

• The greatest risk for a hypoglycemic reaction is during the sleep-time fast between dinner and breakfast, and before a meal or snack time.

• Changes in insulin doses, or changes in meal plans, should be closely supervised and monitored by the nurse and the physician.

Most diabetic diets are based on the exchange program of the American Diabetes and American Dietetic Associations, and the ideal body weight, metabolic rate, and activity level of each individual diabetic client. Usually, the diet is 60 percent carbohydrate, 20 percent protein, and 20 percent fat in three daily meals and a nighttime snack. Simple and refined sugars should be avoided abut may be substituted with artificial sweeteners. Diabetic clients must be taught to carefully read food labels to determine that foods are "sugar-free." Figure 8–2 shows an example of a food label.

Nutrition Facts	
Serving Size: 1/2 Cup	
Servings Per Container: 4	

Amount Per Serving	
Calories 100 Calories from Fat 30	
	% Daily Value*
Total Fat 3g	**5%**
Saturated Fat 0g	**0%**
Cholesterol 0mg	**0%**
Sodium 340mg	**14%**
Total Carbohydrate 15g	**5%**
Dietary Fiber 1g	**4%**
Sugars 0g	
Protein 2g	

Vitamin A 0% • Vitamin C 0%
Calcium   0%   •   Iron   2%

*Percent Daily Values are based on a 2,000 calorie diet. Your daily values may be higher or lower depending on your calorie needs:

	Calories	2,000	2,500
Total Fat	Less than	65g	80g
Sat Fat	Less than	20g	25g
Cholesterol	Less than	300mg	300mg
Sodium	Less than	2,400mg	2,400mg
Total Carbohydrate		300g	375g
Dietary Fiber		25g	30g

Calories per gram:
Fat 9 • Carbohydrate 4 • Protein 4

Ingredients: Flour, Water, Yeast Vegetable Oil, Salt, Artificial Flavor and Color.

● **Figure 8–2** Labels on food packages give facts about the ingredients and nutrition of the food in the package.

The amount of food ingested is dependent on the client's height, weight, body size, age, gender, and activity level. Caloric requirement is based on the need for energy to maintain the client's desirable body weight. The formula for figuring the percentage of fat is:

Percent of calories from fat = $\dfrac{\text{Grams of fat per serving} \times 9}{\text{Total calories per serving}}$

An example of a diabetic diet is:
2000 Calories

Protein:	2000 x .15 = 300 Calories
	$\dfrac{300 \text{ Calories}}{4 \text{ calories/g}}$ = 75 g Protein
Carbohydrate:	2000 x .60 = 1200 Calories
	$\dfrac{1200 \text{ Calories}}{4 \text{ calories/g}}$ = 300 g Carbohydrates
Fat:	2000 x .25 = 500 Calories
	$\dfrac{500 \text{ Calories}}{9 \text{ calories/g}}$ = 55 g Fat

Diabetic clients are told exactly what they should eat. Any special dietary considerations such as weight reduction or cholesterol restriction should be by the direction of a nutritionist. All individuals involved in diet planning, purchasing of food, and preparation of meals should be kept up to date for all diet changes made by the nutritionist. Figure 8–3 shows the food pyramid which illustrates how a balanced diet is conceived.

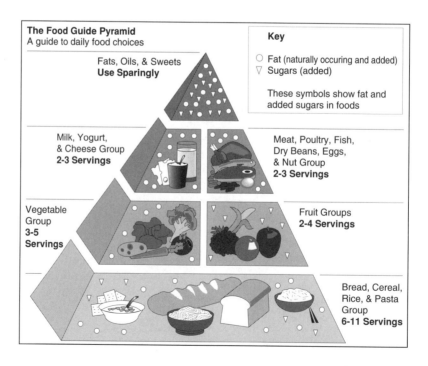

Figure 8–3 The food pyramid shows how to build a balanced diet. (Courtesy: U.S. Department of Agriculture).

complex carbohydrates come from starch sources and are slow to be changed to blood glucose.

simple carbohydrates come from sugar souces and are quickly changed to blood glucose.

Most nutritionists prefer diabetic diets incorporate **complex carbohydrates** rather than **simple carbohydrates**. These include:

Simple carbohydrates

- Sucrose (white or brown table sugar) and foods that contain large quantities of sugar such as jams, jellies, candy, and sugar-sweetened beverages.
- Fructose in fruit or as sweeteners
- Honey, syrups, molasses, and corn syrup.

Complex Carbohydrates

- Grains wheat, oats, corn, rye, barley, and rice.
- Foods made from grains cereals, breads, and pastas.
- Certain vegetables such as potatoes, sweet peas, dried beans, and lentils.

The HCA observes and evaluates the client and/or family demonstrate compliance and understanding of the diet. This includes purchasing and preparing the proper food.

Purchasing proper foods is the result of careful information and guidelines, and reading the food labels. Today's market has a vast variety of foods appropriate to diabetic diets, and the new labeling law requires extensive nutritional data be included in the labels such as serving size, fat and carbohydrate content, sodium and vitamin content, and calorie content.

Alcohol contributes 7 kilocalories per gram and must be avoided in the total daily dietary regime. Alcohol also elevates blood glucose, but later causes a drop by inhibiting hepatic glucose production. Diabetics should avoid alcohol, but if they do drink, they should not do so on an empty stomach.

In preparing meals, the amount of fat and/or sugar used is vital. Alternative sweeteners such as Equal™ or SweetOne™ can be substituted for sugar. Recipes for cooking food under diabetic rules are easily available. A well-balanced, nutritious diet which complies to physician guidelines is the goal of diet management in home care. The home is the perfect setting for the aide to observe the diet plan. Figure 8–4 shows a well-balanced meal.

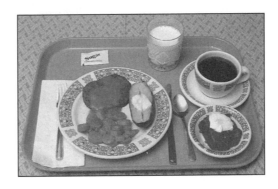

Figure 8–4 Well-balanced, smaller servings are more appealing to the elderly appetite.

But what about when the patient is ill? We have mentioned that illness and/or stress can affect blood glucose levels. The physician should be notified of colds, flu, fever, or infections in the diabetic clients so that more frequent blood glucose monitoring can be ordered. The need for insulin will increase, even if there is less food eaten. Many people mistakenly assume that if they are ill and unable to eat, they should not take their insulin. At these times it is important to check blood sugar levels, and adjust insulin dosages as ordered by the physician.

The client's wellness depends on his or her active participation. HCAs are the one constant influence on his or her acceptance and cooperation, so look on this as a welcome challenge.

COMPLICATIONS

Complications occur frequently in the client with diabetes as the illness progresses. These complications have been discussed in terms of chronic and acute complications in Chapter 5 and 6. However, in terms of client education, it is extremely important that the client and family understand the signs and symptoms of each complication in order for them to be prevented. There are some complications that simply occur as a result of the disease. The important aspect in client education is for the client to recognize the first signs and symptoms so that the complications can be treated in the early stages before they become irreversible. The acute complications the nurse teaches the client include hypoglycemia, hyperglycemia, insulin shock, ketoacidosis, and foot complications. The chronic complications covered by client education include vascular problems, eye disorders, neuropathy, infections, skin integrity, and chronic stress.

Preventing a hypoglycemic attack can often be achieved by the HCA, the nurse, and the physician by teaching the client remedies to balance a possible insulin reaction. Changing the carbohydrate level of the diet to match the situation is one such remedy. Table 8–3 shows some examples of when to change the carbohydrate level of the diet.

Table 8–3 When to Change the Client's Carbohydrate Level		
Situation	**Remedy**	**Adjust Meal?**
Insulin Reaction	10 g carbohydrate. If lasting more than 15 minutes, take more carbohydrates	No
Light Exercise	Do not increase carbohydrates	No
Moderate Exercise	10–15 g carb./hr. of exercise	No
Vigorous Exercise	20–30 g carb./hr. of exercise	No
Delayed Meal	15–30 g. carbs. will prevent reaction every 6–8 hrs	Yes—Deduct the carb. from the meal
Illness	50–75 g. carbs. every 6–8 hrs.	Replaces the meal

EXERCISE

The effects of exercise sometimes create situations in which insulin reactions result. The three important factors in exercise are that it is consistent, there are planned rest periods, and there is awareness of how it affects blood glucose levels. To determine these three factors, the HCA may be involved in observing the client's individual physical tolerance level. Exercise is beneficial to improve cardiovascular circulation, fat levels, blood pressure control, emotional well-being, muscle tone and flexibility, bone density, metabolism, and glucose tolerance. The benefits of exercise are many, but it is important for the client to have a safe exercise plan so negative effects such as hyperglycemia, ketosis, and unstable metabolism do not occur.

aerobic exercises are done to increase the heart rate and provide increased oxygen and improved circulation to the body.

Aerobic exercises includes walking, jogging, swimming, biking, and dancing. Aerobic exercise is the most helpful in glycemic control. Before beginning an exercise program, the client must first have a physician's approval.

The following are examples of exercise programs that may be approved by the physician for each type of diabetic.

Diabetics—Type I

Exercise: Any aerobic exercise.

Duration: As long as there are no complications

Diabetics—Type II (obese)

Exercise: Low-impact exercises such as walking, biking, and swimming; *no* running.

Duration: 30 minutes to 1 hour

Diabetics—Type II (non-obese)

Exercise: Low-impact exercises such as walking, biking, and swimming; *no* running.

Duration: 20 to 30 minutes.

Exercising seven days a week if possible is generally recommended for both Type I and Type II diabetes. This consistency makes it easier for the client to balance medications and meals. The following five guidelines are recommended:

1. Clients with diabetes should exercise, if possible, 30 minutes to $1^1/_2$ hours after meals to avoid low blood glucose and prevent high blood glucose levels after meals.

2. Clients with diabetes should try to avoid peak insulin times, and avoid using the limb which is the site of injection.

3. Clients with diabetes should avoid exercising within 60 minutes of an injection of regular insulin.

4. Clients with diabetes should always carry glucose tablets or another source of quick sugar, wear an ID bracelet, carry an ID card, and if possible, exercise with another person.

5. clients with diabetes should monitor their blood glucose levels right before exercising and again 30 minutes after exercising. If the client is new to an exercise program, more frequent monitoring should be done, and if glucose levels are 240mg/dl, ketones should be checked. If moderate ketones are present, exercise should stop until more professional advise is given. Client should not exercise if blood glucose is greater than 300.

    Diabetic clients should be aware that exercise may create a need for less medication and/or an increase in foods before, during, and after they exercise.

    If the client has complications such as retinopathy, nephropathy, or hypertension, he or she should be closely monitored by a physician and/or exercise physiologist. Exercise is healthy for your diabetic clients, but the HCA must play a role in observation and evaluation to keep that client healthy and safe.

SOCIAL SUPPORT

Social support of the client and family is important for the client with diabetes. Social support comes from outside the home, such as extended family, churches, neighbors, and clubs. These social supports may be the difference between a happy and cooperative client and one who is isolated, depressed, and who does not care about his or her own well-being. The HCA may be the only support person the client has. For clients with diabetes who live alone, the medical social worker (MSW) may need to be called in on the case to assess the situation and make recommendations for more client support. These may include support groups in the community, meal services, homemakers, or home maintenance persons.

The nurse or MSW may asses the family system for its value as a support for the client. This is especially important for the elderly client with diabetes and for children with diabetes. Some questions to assess the level of support provided by the family include:

*   How involved is the family in the daily care of the client?
*   What type of relationship does the family and client have? Is it flexible or rigid, loving or abusive, accepting or neglectful?
*   Is the client encouraged to do as much for himself or herself as possible, or is the client's dependency on others encouraged?
*   Who is available for this client's support? Are there children, grandchildren, brothers, sisters, or a spouse living in the home?
*   How well is the client adapting to the illness psychologically?

- How many lifestyle changes has the client and family had to make?
- What are the family's personal beliefs about the disease?
- How motivated is the family to being supportive?

REVIEW QUESTIONS

1. The education of the client and family is the responsibility of the _____.
2. A trained and educated expert on diabetic diet management is a _____.
3. A time delay for meals of not more than _____ is appropriate for diabetics.
4. Diabetics should always carry _____.
5. _____ is a morning rise in glucose due to insulin sensitivity.
6. Which of the following is not an example of 10 to 15 grams of rapid-acting carbohydrates?
    a. 2 ounces diet soda
    b. 3 graham crackers
    c. 2 tablespoons of raisins
    d. 8 ounces milk
7. The greatest risk of a hypoglycemic episode occurs:
    a. during sleep time
    b. before meals
    c. before snack time
    d. all of the above
8. Which is the usual ADA diet?
    a. 40% carbohydrate, 40% protein, 20% fat
    b. 60% carbohydrate, 30% protein, 10% fat
    c. 60% carbohydrate, 20% protein, 20% fat
    d. 40% carbohydrate, 50% protein, 10% fat
9. Examples of simple carbohydrates include:
    a. honey and corn syrup
    b. breads and pastas
    c. peas and beans
    d. all of the above
10. The best advice for diabetics on drinking alcohol is:
    a. calculate 9 kilograms per gram into the diet
    b. alcohol always elevates blood glucose
    c. avoid it
    d. drink on an empty stomach
11. True or False? Stress effects the client's glucose levels.

12. True or False? The flu can effect the client's glucose levels.
13. True or False? Infections can effect the client's glucose levels.
14. Unscramble the following key term from the chapter: xmcpeol rtabyescodarh _____
    _____

Safety and Emergencies

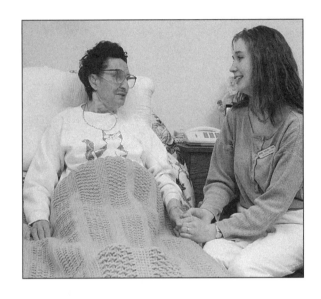

OBJECTIVES

Upon reading this chapter and completing the review questions, the HCA should be able to:

1. Understand safety and emergency situations.
2. Observe the client's environment in terms of safety measures.
3. Name the most common safety hazards in the home.
4. List some conditions that promote safety and prevent falls.
5. State some basic facts of medication safety.
6. Be familiar with emergency measures in home care.
7. Demonstrate an understanding of positioning the client and transfer safety.
8. Recognize safety and emergency situations specific to care of the client with diabetes.

KEY TERMS

aseptic
confused
disoriented
flammable

infection
pathogen
safe environment

INTRODUCTION

safe environment an environment free of hazards to prevent illness or injury.

The home can be an unsafe area for the homebound client as well as for the HCA who cares for that client. Clients who are ill and weak are more prone to accidents at home, and are usually unable to handle an emergency.

Safety is one of the HCA's responsibilities. He or she can create a **safe environment** for the client by preventing, correcting, or eliminating conditions that cause accidents and assist the client and family with measures to prepare for crisis intervention.

All clients cared for in the home have the right to a healthy and safe environment. When caring for the client with diabetes who has poor judgment or is unsteady, the hazards are greater. Therefore, the responsibilities for client safety are increased, and the caregiver becomes the person who truly safeguards the client. The nurse on the case assesses the home for safety because the potential for injury to these persons is greater than for the average client.

Falls are the leading cause of death or injury in persons over the age of 65. The client with diabetes who falls and becomes injured himself is an even greater nursing challenge because of their impaired healing ability.

OBSERVING FOR POTENTIAL RISKS

The potential for injury is especially high for the client with diabetes. When observing for potential risks, the HCA should consider the following:

- the client's level of function
- the client's emotional state
- incontinence
- the use of medications
- poor eyesight
- poor hearing
- balance problems
- any history of alcohol use
- history of falls

The HCA is responsible for keeping the home environment safe and free from hazards. It is important to review some of the basic safety rules and apply them to the situation when caring for a client with diabetes. Some general safety measures for clients in the home include:

- No smoking allowed unless someone stays with the client every minute; matches should be locked away.
- Electrical cords off the floor and out of sight.
- Loose rugs removed.

- Stairs, halls, and doorways kept free of clutter.
- Furniture arranged to allow free movement.
- Grab bars installed in the bathtub, shower, and toilet area.
- Nonskid rubber mats placed in the bathtub and shower.
- A first aid kit kept in the home at all times.
- Smoke alarm and fire extinguishers in good working order.
- All medicine locked away.
- Nonskid soles on shoes worn by the client.
- All hazardous tools and firearms locked away.
- Emergency numbers in easy access of the telephone (Figure 9–1). The HCA should discuss emergency communications with the family and report to the supervisor if problems exist.
- Nightlights provided everywhere in the home.
- The temperature of the hot water heater lowered to prevent problems when there is no one around.
- Poisons locked away.

Helpful Hints: Never leave clients alone when they are bathing or showering. The HCA should always be close by, and check the client frequently.

The bathroom can be a potentially hazardous area and the following should be considered:

- The toilet seat should be secure.
- Have a spare key in another part of the house if the door has a lock.
- The client should be able to get on and off the toilet safely.
- Hot and cold water faucets should be correctly marked.
- Floors should never be wet and slippery.

The kitchen area also can be especially dangerous for the client with diabetes. The following safety guidelines are specific for the kitchen area:

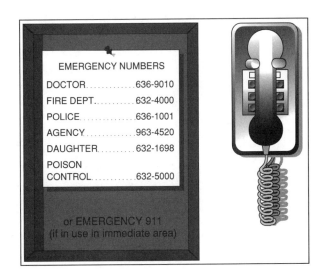

EMERGENCY NUMBERS

DOCTOR 636-9010

FIRE DEPT 632-4000

POLICE 636-1001

AGENCY 963-4520

DAUGHTER 632-1698

POISON
CONTROL 632-5000

or EMERGENCY 911
(if in use in immediate area)

Figure 9–1 Important numbers posted next to the telephone may save precious moments during an emergency. Check your local directory for the correct numbers.

- The kitchen should have a fire extinguisher and a smoke alarm in good working order.
- The handles of pans should be turned toward the back of the stove when in use.
- Grease and liquids should be thoroughly cleaned when spillage occurs, especially on the floor.
- Cleaning liquids such as polishes, bleaches, and detergents should be kept locked away.
- Sharp knives should be kept in a locked drawer.
- An escape plan should be created and posted in the kitchen with an exit route established in case of fire.
- Always read labels of bleaches, detergents, and chemicals; never combine these because noxious gases could result.
- Arrange items frequently used by the client within his or her reach to prevent clients from falls caused by climbing.

The HCA should observe the home for safety at every visit. A safety checklist should be kept on the client's record, and a weekly review done by the nurse and/or the HCA. The safety recommendations should be placed in a prominent place so that all family members and caregivers can refer to it easily.

MAINTAINING A SAFE ENVIRONMENT IN THE HOME

When the client is admitted to home health care, the skilled nurse does a safety assessment of the home during the admission process. A safety checklist is usually included in the admission packet, as safety measures and interventions begin at that time. The HCA follows up on this process. The nurse includes the client's family, and the rest of the healthcare team, when setting safety goals, and determining if the goals have been met. The HCA should constantly assess the quality of the environment and look for safety hazards. If any are discovered, the HCA should report them to the supervisor immediately.

A safe environment is one in which a person has a low risk of illness or injury. Some elderly and frail persons cannot assume the responsibility for their own safety. Poor vision may play a part in your client's inability to be safe at home. This could lead to falls, tripping, and misreading labels. Hearing loss is another factor affecting the client's safety as warning signals, such as fire detectors, may not be heard.

The most common safety hazards in the home are:

- Damaged electrical wiring on large and small appliances or overloaded electrical outlets (Figure 9–2A and B)
- Faulty or uneven stairs

Helpful Hints: The agency is responsible for the client's safety. Therefore, the HCA, as the agency's representative, is also responsible.

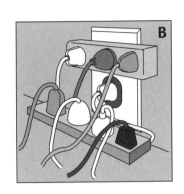

Figure 9–2 (A) Electrical cords in an unsafe condition. (B) There are too many plugs in this outlet.

flammable able to catch fire.

- Loose rugs that slip (Figure 9–3)
- Poisons
- **Flammable** cleaning rags, mops, and brooms
- Sharp objects such as knives, razors, and lawn tools
- Wet floors
- Cluttered hallways
- Unstable furniture

Falls

Falls are the most common accidents in the home, particularly among the elderly. Most falls occur in the bedroom or bathroom, and are caused by slippery floors, throw rugs, poor lighting, cluttered floors, furniture that is out of place, or slippery bathtubs and showers. Some conditions that promote safety and prevent falls are:

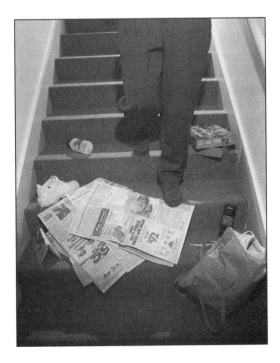

Figure 9–3 Cluttered stairways are hazardous for elderly clients who have difficulty with vision or balance.

1. Adequate lighting in rooms and hallways.
2. Hand rails on both sides of stairs, in halls, and in bathrooms.
3. Carpeting tacked down and throw rugs avoided.
4. Nonskid shoes and slippers worn by clients when walking.
5. Nonskid waxes used on hardwood, tiled, or linoleum floors.
6. Floors uncluttered with toys and other objects.
7. Electrical cords and extension cords kept out of the path of the client.
8. Furniture left in place and not rearranged.
9. A telephone and lamp placed at the bedside.
10. Nonskid bathmats in tubs and showers (Figure 9–4).
11. Weak clients assisted when walking, getting out of bed, getting out of the tub or shower, and with other activities ordered by the physician.
12. A call bell within easy reach.
13. Cracked steps, loose hand rails, and frayed carpets reported and repaired promptly.
14. Frequently used items placed within the client's easy reach.
15. The bed in the low position to minimize the distance from the bed to the floor if the client falls or gets out of bed.
16. Night lights in the client's room and hallways kept on at night.
17. Floors kept free of spills and excess furniture.
18. Crutches, canes, and walkers must have nonskid tips.
19. Wheels on beds and wheelchairs locked when transferring clients.

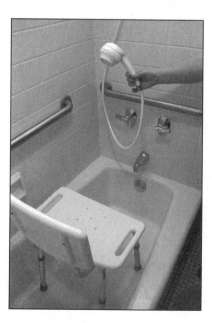

Figure 9–4 Safety features for the tub include several types of bars and nonskid strips that allow clients to get into and out of the tub safely.

20. Gates at the tops and bottoms of stairs when there are infants and toddlers in the home (the child should not be able to put his or her head through the gate bars).
21. Side rails installed on the client's bed, if possible.

Medication Safety

Storage and disposal of medications in the home are major problems for home health workers. HCAs should never dispense or administer medication. However, the HCA needs information about certain medications because many clients receiving home care services are taking them. HCAs often hand medications to their clients, remind clients to take medications, and report their use, misuse, and effects to their supervisors.

Safety guidelines for medications include:

1. When cleaning the medicine cabinet, special care should be taken not to disturb medication container labels.
2. Medication containers should be replaced in the same position in the medicine cabinet after cleaning, because clients expect a bottle to be in one position and do not look at the label.
3. If more than one person in the household is taking medications, keep the medications in separate rooms to avoid a client from taking the wrong medication.
4. Encourage the client to dispose of old medications correctly by flushing them down the toilet, and report the disposal to the supervisor.
5. The client should store medications in a specific area and tell the family members where it is. The medications should not be moved.
6. Know if there are special instructions for storage of medications, such as refrigeration.
7. Never refer to medications as candy.
8. Never add medication from one bottle to another, even if it is labeled as the same medication. This is considered dispensing medication, and the expiration dates could be different.
9. Never break, crush, or alter the form of the medication in any way.

The five "rights" for medication safety are:

- The *right* client
- The *right* medication
- The *right* time
- The *right* way to take the medication (oral, etc.)
- The *right* dose

Helpful Hints: Keep your eyes and ears open for over-the-counter medication use and misuse that should be reported to the nurse and/or supervisor.

EMERGENCY MEASURES IN HOME CARE

HCAs may be called on to handle emergency situations in the home. All HCAs should have a basic first aid course. Figure 9–5 shows first aid procedures in case of a fire.

There are two emergency situations in diabetes:

1. Insulin shock—if the client has too much insulin.

2. Diabetic coma—if the client does not have enough insulin.

It is important for the HCA to understand both of these emergency situations, the causes, and the signs of symptoms of each (see Chapter 5).

> **Helpful Hints:** All HCAs should keep current on the symptoms of these two emergency situations, and post them in the home where all members of the health care team, the client, and the family can refer to them.

First Aid: What to do in a Fire Emergency	
What to Do	**Escape Plan**

If you catch on fire:
Don't panic and don't run.
Running increases the flames.
Instead:
1. **Stop.**
2. **Drop** to the ground.
3. **Roll.** Continue to roll until you have completely put out the fire.
4. Remove clothing from the affected area. *Do not* attempt to remove clothing that sticks.
5. Flush area with cool water.
6. Cover with a sterile pad or clean sheet.
7. *Seek immediate medical attention.*
 	
If the burn is from a chemical:
1. Follow steps 4–7 above and flush with cool water for 20-30 minutes.
2. If the eyes are involved, flush them for at least 20 minutes or until medical help arrives.
3. Remove contact lenses.
 	
If the burn is electrical:
1. Turn off electrical source before touching victim.
2. Check for breathing and pulse. If absent, start Cardiopulmonary Resuscitation (CPR), if qualified.
3. Follow steps 4–7 above.
	• Develop a Family Escape Plan
	• Include two exits from each room.
	• Plan a meeting place outside the home.
	• Practice the plan.
	
	Plan of Escape: Evacuate!
	Do not attempt to fight the fire.
	1. If in bed, roll off onto the floor.
	2. Stay low! Crawl if necessary. Smoke rises, and oxygen will remain near the floor.
	3. Cover your mouth and nose with some clothing or material to aid in breathing.
	4. Place your hands on any closed door before opening it. If it is hot, *do not open it!* Find another exit. If it is not hot, open it slowly, standing to the side. *Do not use elevators.*
	5. *If you are trapped in a room:*
	  a. Roll a rug or other material and place across the bottom of the door.
	  b. Open a window, both top and bottom, to allow air to enter and smoke to escape.
	  c. Telephone for help, if possible.
	  d. Attract attention; call for help.

For further information, call The Burn Center at New York Hospital-Cornell Medical Center, 535 East 68th Street, New York, NY, at (212)-472-6890.	

Figure 9–5 What to do in a fire emergency.

Emergency Plans

Each emergency situation is different. The following rules apply to all kinds of emergency:

1. HCAs should know their limitations and not try a procedure that is unfamiliar.

2. HCAs should remain calm at all times. Being calm helps the victim feel more secure.

3. HCAs should observe the client for life-threatening problems by checking breathing, pulse, and for bleeding.

4. HCAs should keep the victim lying down or in the position which he or she was found, and should *never* move the victim. Moving a victim could make the injury worse.

5. HCAs should perform necessary emergency measures.

6. HCAs should call for help or instruct someone to call 911. An operator will send emergency vehicles and personnel to the scene. The person calling 911 should give the following information to the operator:

   - The location, including the street address, and city or town.
   - The telephone number where the victim is.
   - What happened (a fall, for example) since fire equipment, police, and ambulances may be needed.
   - How many people require emergency medical attention.
   - The conditions of the victims, any obvious injuries, and if there is a life-threatening situation.
   - The aid currently being given.

7. HCAs should not remove any clothing unless absolutely necessary.

8. The victim should be kept warm. Aides can cover the victim with a blanket or a coat.

9. HCAs should reassure the conscious victim by explaining what is happening, and that help has been called.

10. HCAs should not give the victim any foods or fluids.

11. HCAs should keep onlookers away from the victim to maintain the victim's privacy.

Every home should have a plan in case of emergencies (Figure 9–6). However, the home with an elderly, frail, ill, or impaired person must take extra measures to plan ahead for emergency situations.

Reporting an accident or emergency by phone should be done in a calm manner. It is important to have emergency phone numbers written next to the telephone(s). This list should include:

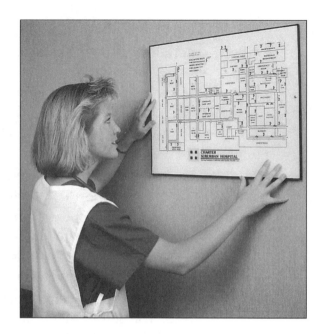

Figure 9–6 Client and family should know the escape plan in the event of a fire.

- Emergency Medical Service (often 911), if available
- Police department
- Fire department
- Responsible family member at work
- The home care supervisor and agency
- Client's physician
- Nearest hospital
- Ambulance service (if different from 911)
- Poison control center
- If there is no telephone in the client's home, arrange in advance to use a neighbor's in case of emergency

Fire Safety

There are three major causes of fires in this country: faulty electrical equipment and wiring, overloaded electrical circuits, and smoking. Fire safety measures include:

1. Following the fire safety precautions for the use of oxygen.
2. Making sure all ashes, cigar, and cigarette butts are out before emptying ashtrays.
3. Providing ashtrays to clients who are allowed to smoke.
4. Emptying ashtrays into metal containers partly filled with sand or water. Do not empty ashtrays into wastebaskets or plastic containers lined with paper or plastic bags.
5. Supervising the smoking client who cannot protect himself or herself. This includes **confused**, **disoriented**, and sedated clients.

confused disturbed orientation to time, place and person.

disoriented a state of mental confusion as to time, place, and identity.

6. Following the safety practices for using electrical equipment.

7. Supervising the play of children, and keeping matches out of their reach.

If three elements are present in the right proportions, a fire will result (Figure 9–7). The three elements are heat, fuel and oxygen.

The following guidelines will help the HCA protect the client if there is a fire. The HCA should:

- call the fire department (have fire emergency numbers near the client's telephones.
- plan escape routes from each room.
- know where fire extinguishers are and how to use them.
- know where fire alarms boxes are located
- turn off any oxygen or electrical equipment in the general area of the fire
- get the client and others out of the house
- try to fight a small fire, but leave right away if the fire is out of control.
- close doors if the home is vacated.
- crawl, keeping the client's head close to the floor if the area is filled with smoke.
- cover his or her face with a damp cloth or towel in a smoke-filled area.
- feel any doors before they are opened, and do not open a door that feels hot or if smoke is coming from around it.
- when opening a cool door, open it slowly, keeping the head to the side. Doors should be closed immediately if smoke or heat rushes in.

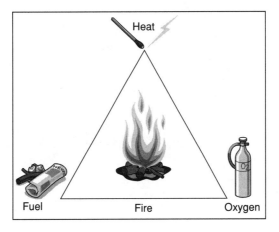

Figure 9–7 The fire triangle shows the elements needed for combustion (burning).

• stuff blankets, clothes, towels, linens, coats, or other cloth at the bottom of the door if the client is trapped inside. A window should be opened for air and a piece of cloth should be hung outside the window to attract attention.

The HCA should be able to use a fire extinguisher (Figure 9–8A and B. Local fire departments often give demonstrations on how to operate a fire extinguisher, and some agencies require all employees to demonstrate how to use one.

The RACE system is used as a general guideline in fire safety (Figure 9–9).

• Remove the clients in immediate danger.

• Activate the alarm (or call the fire department) to alert others.

• Confine the fire by closing doors.

• Extinguish the fire, if possible.

Figure 9–10 shows an HCA protecting a client while escaping from a fire.

> **Helpful Hints:** Do not forget that the escape of a disabled or elderly client is slower than others.

INFECTION CONTROL

> **infection**   illness resulting from the entrance into the body of a pathogen through ingestion, inhalation, or physical contact

All home health personnel must be careful to use proper measures to control **infection** with all clients. The client with diabetes is at a greater risk for infection than any other client. The specialized HCA should keep current on the latest information to protect the client, the family, other workers, and himself or herself from infection.

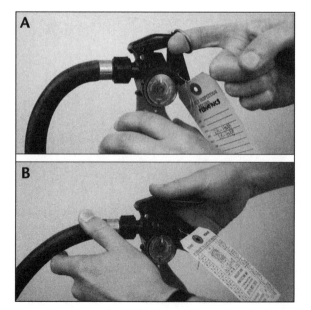

Figure 9–8   The proper use of a fire extinguisher. (A) Remove the pin. (B) Push top handle down.

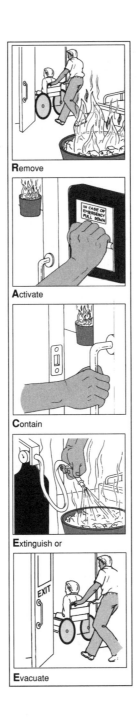

Remove

Activate

Contain

Extinguish or

Evacuate

Figure 9–9 R-A-C-E Procedure.

Universal Precautions

Universal precautions were developed in 1985 by the Centers for Disease Control and Prevention (CDC). These guidelines apply to all healthcare workers for all clients, no matter what the diagnosis is or where they are being cared for. If proper precautions are not taken, **pathogens** can be transmitted by the HCAs to themselves, their families, other clients, and their families by means of skin and clothing. Universal precautions protect against many different types of infections including AIDS, tuberculosis (TB) and Hepatitis B.

pathogens microbes which cause infection.

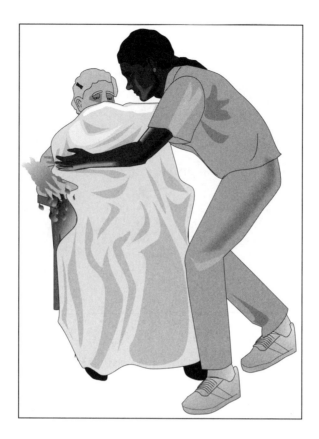

Figure 9–10 An HCA protects the client's face.

Standard Precautions

The CDC published new recommendations in 1996 called standard precautions (Figure 9–11). This new information is based on several years of research and data collection to:

1. Improve the criteria for universal precautions.
2. Change some of the medical terminology.
3. Offer new information on drug resistant pathogens.
4. Update isolation guidelines.

Personal Protective Equipment (PPE)

Personal Protective Equipment provides a barrier between the client and health care worker. When used correctly, PPE provides a barrier that prevents the transfer of pathogens from one person to another. Standard Precautions require all health care workers to wear PPE anytime they expect to have contact with

- blood
- any moist body fluid exccept sweat, secretions or excretions
- mucous membranes
- nonintact skin

STANDARD PRECAUTIONS FOR INFECTION CONTROL

Wash Hands (Plain soap)
Wash after touching blood, body fluids, secretions, excretions, and contaminated items. Wash immediately after gloves are removed and between patient contacts. Avoid transfer of microorganisms to other patients or environments.

Wear Gloves
Wear when touching blood, body fluids, secretions, excretions, and contaminated items. Put on clean gloves just before touching mucous membranes and nonintact skin. Change gloves between tasks and procedures on the same patient after contact with material that may contain high concentrations of microorganisms. Remove gloves promptly after use, before touching noncontaminated items and environmental surfaces, and before going to another patient, and wash hands immediately to avoid transfer of microorganisms to other patients or environments.

Wear Mask and Eye Protection or Face Shield
Protect mucous membranes of the eyes, nose and mouth during procedures and patient-care activities that are likely to generate splashes or sprays of blood, body fluids, secretions, or excretions.

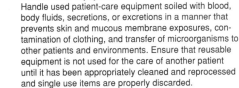

Wear Gown
Protect skin and prevent soiling of clothing during procedures that are likely to generate splashes or sprays of blood, body fluids, secretions, or excretions. Remove a soiled gown as promptly as possible and wash hands to avoid transfer of microorganisms to other patients or environments.

Patient-Care Equipment
Handle used patient-care equipment soiled with blood, body fluids, secretions, or excretions in a manner that prevents skin and mucous membrane exposures, contamination of clothing, and transfer of microorganisms to other patients and environments. Ensure that reusable equipment is not used for the care of another patient until it has been appropriately cleaned and reprocessed and single use items are properly discarded.

Environmental Control
Follow hospital procedures for routine care, cleaning, and disinfection of environmental surfaces, beds, bedrails, bedside equipment and other frequently touched surfaces.

Linen
Handle, transport, and process used linen soiled with blood, body fluids, secretions, or excretions in a manner that prevents exposure and contamination of clothing, and avoids transfer of microorganisms to other patients and environments.

Occupational Health and Bloodborne Pathogens
Prevent injuries when using needles, scalpels, and other sharp instruments or devices; when handling sharp instruments after procedures; when cleaning used instruments; and when disposing of used needles.

Never recap used needles using both hands or any other technique that involves directing the point of a needle towards any part of the body; rather, use either a one-handed "scoop" technique or a mechanical device designed for holding the needle sheath.

Do not remove used needles from disposable syringes by hand, and do not bend, break, or otherwise manipulate used needles by hand. Place used disposable syringes and needles, scalpels, blades, and other sharp items in puncture-resistant sharps containers located as close as practical to the area in which the items were used, and place reusable syringes and needles in a puncture-resistant container for transport to the reprocessing area.

Use resuscitation devices as an alternative to mouth-to-mouth resuscitation.

Patient Placement
Use a private room for a patient who contaminates the environment or who does not (or cannot be expected to) assist in maintaining appropriate hygiene or environmental control. Consult Infection Control if a private room is not available.

Figure 9–11 Standard Precautions (Courtesy: BREVIS Corporation, Salt Lake City, UT).

PPE includes gloves, water resistant gowns, face shields or masks and goggles. HCAs should follow their agency policies for use of PPE in routine tasks.

Some medical terms associated with infection control include:

Visible: able to be seen with the eye

Body Substance Isolation: precautions requiring special handling of all fluids

Drug Resistant: disease-causing organisms that resist treatment with normal antibiotics

Reservoir: a human being who has an infection that can be spread to others.

Airborne Transmission: tiny microbes spread in the air over long distances such as TB.

Droplet Transmission: disease spread by respiratory secretions or droplets in the air within a distance of three feet.

Transmission-Based Precautions: CDC recommendations for isolating clients in addition to standard precautions.

Table 9–1 lists the disease requiring transmission-based precautions.

Higher-Efficiency Particulate Air Mask (HEPA): a special mask with tiny pores to prevent airborne transmissions.

Pathogens, which are the cause of infections, can be controlled with good cleaning techniques and maintenance. It is important to keep an **aseptic** environment for the client. Some common aseptic practices are:

aseptic free of germs

- Washing hands before and after touching the client.
- Washing hands after urinating, having a bowel movement, or changing tampons or sanitary napkins.
- Washing hands before handling or preparing food.
- Washing fruits and vegetables before serving them.
- Encouraging each family member to use his or her own towels, washcloths, toothbrush, drinking glass, and other personal care items.

Table 9–1   Diseases Requiring Transmission-Based Isolation Precautions

Disease or Condition	Type of Precautions
AIDS	Standard (or reverse if facility policy)
Chickenpox	Airborne and Contact
Diarrhea	Standard
Drug-resistant skin infections	Contact
German measles	Droplet
Head or body lice	Contact
Hepatitis, type A	Standard. Use contact if diarrhea or incontinent patient
Hepatitis, other types	Standard
HIV disease	Standard
Impetigo	Contact
Infected pressure sore with no drainage	Standard
Infected pressure sore with heavy drainage	Contact
Infectious diarrehea caused by a known pathogen	Contact
Measles	Airborne
Mumps	Droplet
Oral or genital herpes	Standard
Scabies	Contact
Syphilis	Standard
Tuberculosis of the lungs	Airborne
Widespread shingles	Airborne and Contact

Use standard precautions in addition to other types of precautions listed.

- Using disposable cups and dishes for clients with an infection.
- Encouraging the client to cover the nose and mouth with tissues when coughing, sneezing, or blowing their nose. Make sure there is a plastic or paper bag for used tissues.
- Practicing good personal hygiene. Bathe, wash hair, and brush teeth regularly.
- Encouraging clients to wash their hands often. They should wash their hands after toileting and before eating.
- Washing cooking and eating utensils with soap and water after they have been used.
- Cleaning cooking and eating surfaces with soap and water or a disinfectant.
- Not leaving food sitting out and uncovered. Close all food containers, and refrigerate foods that will spoil.
- Not using food that smells bad or looks discolored.
- Checking the expiration date on food. Do not use it if the date has passed.
- Changing water in flower vases daily.
- Removinging dead plants and flowers from the home.
- Dusting furniture with a damp cloth and using a damp mop on floors. This helps prevent the movement of dust in the air.
- Emptying garbage every day. Use large, sturdy plastic bags or wrap the garbage in several thicknesses of newspaper. Place the garbage outside the home. If possible, put the bags in plastic or metal garbage containers.
- Wearing disposable gloves if there are open cuts or sores on hands.
- Holding equipment and linens away from uniform.
- Not shaking linens. This helps prevent the movement of dust.
- Cleaning from the cleanest area to the dirtiest. This prevents soiling a clean area.
- Cleaning away from the body and uniform. Dusting, brushing, or wiping toward oneself transmits microorganisms to the skin, hair, and uniform.
- Pouring contaminated liquids directly into sinks or toilets. Avoid splashing the liquid onto other areas.
- Not sitting on the client's bed, if the client has an infection, to prevent picking up microorganisms and carrying them to the next surface.
- Wearing disposable gloves because the potential for infection in these persons is greater than the average client.
- Wearing a disposable apron when in contact with the client's body fluids

REVIEW QUESTIONS

1. A safe environment is defined as _____.
2. Two sensory disabilities that affect the elderly clients safety are:

   a.

   b.
3. The five rights for safety in taking medications are:

   a. The right _____

   b. The right _____

   c. The right _____

   d. The right _____

   e. The right _____
4. Who does the Admission Safety Assessment of the client and the home?

   a. physician

   b. risk manager

   c. nurse

   d. HCA
5. Which of the following are common safety hazards?

   a. wet floors

   b. damaged wiring

   c. poisons

   d. all of the above
6. Which of the following is *not* a HCA responsibility?

   a. safe storage of medications

   b. administering medications

   c. assisting the client with medications

   d. measuring medications
7. True or False? If more than one person in a household is taking medications, the medications should be placed in separate rooms.
8. True or False? Old medications should not be flushed down the toilet.
9. True or False? The HCA should know his or her limitations in emergency situations.
10. True or False? It is never acceptable to cover the client's face with a damp cloth when escaping a smoke-filled room.
11. True or False? The CDC has developed new universal precautions entitled standard precautions.
12. True or False? The HCA can lower the risk of transmission of pathogens by using proper hand-washing procedures.
13. Unscramble the following key term from the chapter: pseacti _____

CHAPTER 10

Abuse

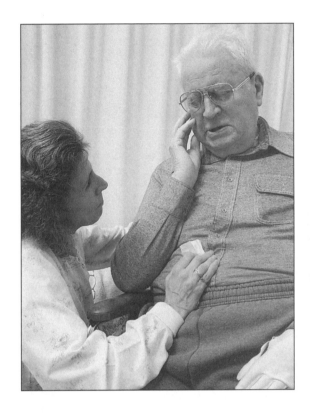

OBJECTIVES

Upon reading this chapter and completing the review questions, the home care aide should be able to:

1. Define the term abuse.
2. Identify six types of abuse and/or neglect.
3. Identify factors contributing to adult abuse.
4. Identify physical indicators of adult abuse, neglect, and exploitation.

KEY TERMS

abuse   intervention
exploitation   self-abuse

INTRODUCTION

Many elderly persons live rich and productive lives with positive relationships with their children and friends. On the other hand, many are severely disabled and live in institutions. Twice that number live with, and are dependent on, their children or siblings. Those elderly persons who are dependent are often a physical, financial, and emotional strain on those persons and families who care for them. Caring for a dependent older adult in the home can cost up to twenty-five thousand dollars per year, and custodial care is *not* a Medicare reimbursable service, and is rarely covered by other health insurance policies. With these two factors common in our society, the 1990s have seen an increase in the neglect and abuse of the elderly population.

abuse the physical or psychological harm inflicted on one person by another. It may or may not be intentional.

Abuse is defined as the infliction of physical pain or injury or any persistent course of conduct intended to produce or result in mental or emotional distress. Severe neglect and severe physical abuse cause great distress and pain, and can lead to injury or death. Figure 10–1 shows a client who may have been abused.

Clients not fully able to care for themselves are easy targets for abuse. This abuse can be administered by untrained, frustrated, or overburdened family members, or by those who deliberately harm others for their own gain.

SIX TYPES OF ABUSE

HCAs are in a position to notice signs of abuse or neglect. If either is occurring, whatever is seen should be handled confidentially. Any signs or abuse or suspicions should be immediately reported to the supervisor.

There are six types of abuse or neglect to watch out for:

1. *Passive Neglect.* Harm is not intended, but occurs because some type of care is not provided because of the caregiver's inability, laziness, or lack of knowledge.

2. *Psychological Abuse.* Harm caused to the client's feeling or emotional state by demeaning, frightening, humiliating, intimidating, isolating, insulting him or her, treating the client as a child, or by using verbal aggression.

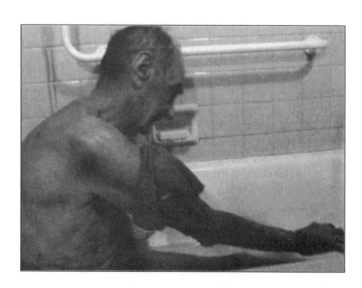

Figure 10–1 Note the bruise on the client's shoulder. The HCA should observe the client, and report any possible signs of abuse to their supervisor.

3. *Material or Financial Abuse.* Stealing, exploiting, or improperly using the client's money, property, or other assets.

4. *Active Neglect.* Intentionally harming the older person physically or psychologically by failing to provide needed care. Examples include deliberately leaving a bed-ridden person alone for lengthy periods, or willfully denying the person food, medication, dentures, or eyeglasses.

5. *Physical Abuse.* Intentionally harming the person physically by such acts as slapping, bruising, sexually molesting, cutting, burning, physically restraining, pushing, or shoving.

6. **Self-Abuse** *or Self-Neglect.* Any of the activities mentioned above committed by the person against himself or herself.

The key is for the HCA to be alert to the physical and mental condition of the client at all times, and to report changes and unusual conditions to the supervisor regularly and promptly.

REPORTING ABUSE

The supervisor must be informed of any suspicions the HCA has in order to identify the proper action to take regarding the reporting of abuse. In order to protect the victim, the situation must be handled carefully; the supervisor and other professionals will become involved if it appears that abuse is taking place.

The primary reasons for not reporting elderly abuse are:

- fear of personal involvement
- lack of evidence that abuse has occurred
- lack of response by authorities
- a generalized belief that reported cases are not satisfactorily handled

Health care providers have a responsibility to report discovered cases of abuse, neglect, or **exploitation**. Forty-one states have laws that mandate the reporting of elder abuse. The law usually states that health professionals or persons who have knowledge of, or who reasonably suspect abuse, must report it. The states also protect the health personnel from civil or criminal liability for the content of the report. Each state has its own laws, and penalties are issued in some states for not reporting abuse.

FACTORS CONTRIBUTING TO ELDERLY ABUSE

The factors contributing to adult abuse include

- **retaliation**
- ageism and violence as a way of life
- lack of close family ties

self-abuse   the injury or pain to which a person subjects himself or herself.

Helpful Hints: It is the law that domestic violence, as well as elderly or child abuse, be reported by health care-givers.

exploitation   a situation in which one person takes unfair advantage of another person.

- lack of community resources
- lack of financial resources
- mental and emotional disorders
- unemployment
- history of alcohol and drug abuse
- environmental conditions
- resentment of dependency
- increased life expectancy
- other situational stresses

SIGNS OF ELDER ABUSE

The three main indicators of adult abuse are:

1. Personal factors, such as ignorance and emotional disturbance.
2. Interpersonal factors, such as unresolved conflicts and lack of gratitude.
3. Situational factors, such as the dependent person living with children and their families, thus causing feeling of frustration and stress to the caregiver(s).

Physical signs of adult (elder) abuse, neglect, or exploitation include:

- the client has unexplained bruises or welts
- the client has unexplained fractures
- the client has unexplained burns
- the client has unexplained lacerations or abrasions
- the client appears mentally confused
- the client has poor personal hygiene
- the client denies being in pain when he or she obviously is
- the client is bedbound, but this is not related to the disease
- the client experiences weight loss
- the client is dehydrated
- the client has old, unexplained scars
- the client is fearful and noncommunicative

Some behavioral signs of abuse are when the client:

- yells obscenities at others
- threatens self-harm or suicide
- refuses medical care
- shows unrealistic fear or hostility
- shows signs of alcohol or drug abuse

- experiences denial of the situation
- stops communicating
- is fearful to be alone (Figure 10–2A)
- cries excessively (Figure 10–2B)
- displays anger at the family
- has a poor self-concept and shows poor self-control
- shows signs of hopelessness

Environmental signs of elderly abuse are:
- The house is dirty and there is garbage around.
- There are fleas, mice, and vermin present in the home.
- The home is overcrowded.
- The home smells of urine or feces.
- The home is not kept at a comfortable temperature.
- The pets are not well cared for.
- There are empty bottles of liquor or medicine containers lying around the home.
- The bed sheets are dirty and have not been changed.
- There is not enough food in the home.
- The food is spoiled and the refrigerator is dirty.
- The food is stored improperly.
- There are no special foods for the client's diet.
- There is no cash available.
- There are unusual withdrawals of money at the bank.
- The client complains of having no money, or that the family is "stealing money."

Helpful Hints: HCAs are in the home more often than any other member of the health care team, and are more likely to be exposed to abusive situations.

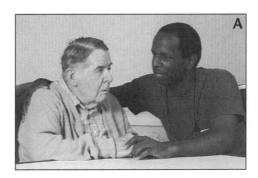

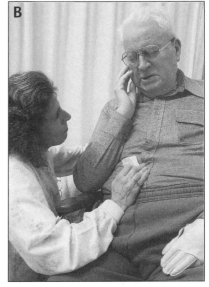

Figure 10–2 Signs of possible behavioral abuse. (A) the client is afraid to be alone. (B) the client experiences excessive crying.

SUBSTANCE ABUSE IN THE ELDERLY

Substance abuse is a causative factor in elder abuse. Abuse of alcohol is a major health problem, and it is the third most common mental disorder in elderly men. Some signs the HCA should look for in clients that may indicate alcoholism are:

- poor personal hygiene
- nutritional problems (weight loss)
- neglect of home
- depression
- suicidal ideas
- repeated falls
- flushed face
- tremors
- extreme fatigue
- incontinence
- withdrawal

Helpful Hints: Confidentiality with peers and family members is important in situations where abuse is suspected or occurring.

intervention interceding on behalf of one person by another.

HCAs should discuss any suspected substance abuse with the supervisor so that the physician can be notified and orders for **intervention** and referral given. The HCA also should observe the client for signs of abuse (Figure 10–3).

PREVENTION

There are a number of ways the HCA can help prevent abuse from starting. Have the client:

- keep a network of friends and activities as long as possible
- participate in community activities

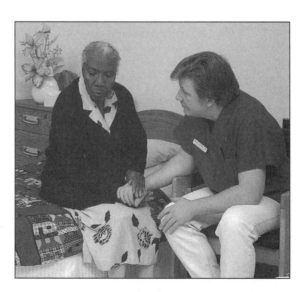

Figure 10–3 The HCA should be especially alert to possible signs of abuse, and report them to the supervisor immediately.

- have a "buddy system" with a friend outside the family and communicate weekly
- make and keep personal care appointments such as dentist and hairdresser
- invite guests to the home frequently
- maintain his or her own telephone
- be neat and organized
- not leave valuables around
- not give up financial control unless it becomes a necessity

REVIEW QUESTIONS

State the type of abuse in each of the following situations:

1. A daughter helps her elderly mother by cashing, depositing, and managing all of her income. All purchases and household bills were made for the mother by the daughter using her mother's checkbook. The daughter, unfortunately, paid her own bills from her mother's account. _____

2. A wife cares for her overweight husband at home after a heart attack. A hospital bed was purchased, but the wife was never instructed to turn the patient or give skin care. She and the neighbor discovered, upon turning the husband three weeks later, that he had developed three large bedsores. _____

3. A couple cared for the wife's elderly mother in their home. The patient was very confused and constantly caused disruptions, so her bedroom was cleared and she was locked in day and night. The couple insisted they did the best they could. The mother was moved to a nursing home, but the couple refused to pay the bill. _____

4. A daughter asked her elderly mother to move in with her soon after her divorce. The daughter began to date, and was away many evenings. The daughter began to resent the mother's verbal concerns. Excessive name-calling and threats to the mother persisted. The mother ran away for three days, but was later returned by the police in a frightened state.
_____

5. An alcoholic son lived with his elderly, sick, and obese mother in her home. She was hospitalized for fractures of the hip and jaw, and bruises to her face and body. The neighbors complained that the son would not allow his mother to leave the house. She died a short time later. Autopsy reports showed that regular beatings had taken place.
_____

6. Which of the following are possible signs of abuse in the elderly?
   a. no access to bank account
   b. poor hygiene
   c. fearfulness
   d. all of the above

7. Behavioral signs of elder abuse include:
   a. bruises and welts
   b. crying and depression
   c. fearfulness
   d. burns
8. True or False? HCAs make a difference in helping a client maintain his or her independence.
9. True or False? The HCA is required by law to report suspected abuse.
10. True or False? A sign of potential abuse is when there is garbage left around the home and the family pets are not well cared for.
11. Unscramble the following key term from the chapter: ronntivieent _____

CHAPTER 11

Psychosocial Influences

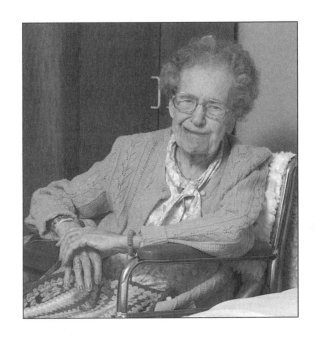

OBJECTIVES

Upon reading this chapter and completing the review questions, the home care aide should be able to:

1. Define psychosocial influences on the client and his or her recovery.
2. Define holistic care of the client with diabetes.
3. Understand multicultural differences and human needs.
4. Describe family dynamics and current changes that may affect the client.
5. Be familiar with positive attitudes and codes of behavior of HCAs.
6. Understand the communication process, especially with the elderly.

KEY TERMS

advocate
confidentiality
culture

family dynamics
holistic caring model
impairment

INTRODUCTION

Most clients receiving home health care live in a family-structured environment. The psycho (emotional) social (human interactions) influences on the client may affect their well-being. The HCA should be aware of these influential factors to better provide the client with a more holistic approach.

THE HOLISTIC MODEL

holistic caring model a treatment method in which physical, emotional, psychological, ethical, and cultural considerations all play a role.

advocate a supporter; one who supports another person.

The **holistic caring model** considers the whole client, including mind, body, spirit, economy, family support, culture, and ethics, and not just the illness or disease process. It also encompasses how these factors affect the recovery of the client (Figure 11–1).

The HCA serves as a client **advocate** (supporter), but cannot be successful without an understanding of the uniqueness and variety of types of clients and families with needs that require special care and concern. Figure 11–2 shows an HCA who is concerned about his client.

The United States has a growing elderly population as well as an increasing multicultural and multiethnic mix. The HCA of the 1990s will be placed in the homes of persons with differences

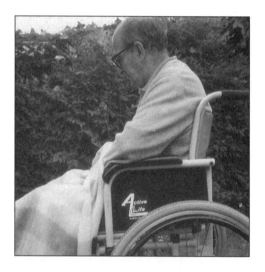

Figure 11–1 Spiritual needs are an important part of caring for the whole client.

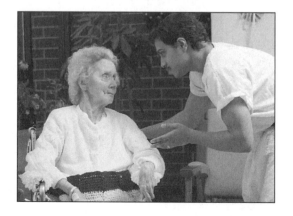

Figure 11–2 The HCA respects differences in clients and families, and understands that each client has needs that require special care and concern.

that could affect the level of care or create barriers to the relationship. Some of the barriers the HCA may see in the home are:

- language differences
- discrimination and distrust
- poverty
- resistance to outside help
- culture bias
- negative attitude toward Western health care
- religious practices
- lack of knowledge of our medical system
- lack of education
- misunderstood family structure

Multicultural differences may occur in race, religion, language, dietary habits, gender, age, culture, economic status, and lifestyle. Table 11–1 shows the differences in dietary practices of certain religions.

One area all humans have in common with each other is their basic needs. A need must be met for a person's well-being. The health caregiver should focus on the client and/or family's needs first, assess the differences, then merge the two to create a care plan for each individual situations. All humans have:

Daily Physical Needs

- food and water
- safety and shelter
- activity and rest
- freedom from pain and discomfort

> **Helpful Hints:** If you believe there is a cultural barrier between you and your client or their family, discuss a change of assignment with your supervisor.

Faith	Christian Science	Roman Catholic	Muslim Moslem	Seventh Day Adventist	Some Baptists	Greek Orthodox (on fast days)
Restricted Food						
Coffee	•			•	•	
Tea	•			•	•	
Alcohol	•		•	•	•	
Pork/pork products			•	•		
Cafeine-containing foods				•		
Dairy products						•
All meats		1 hour before communion; Ash Wed., Good Friday		Small groups		•

Table 11–1 Religious Dietary Practices

In addition, the Jewish Orthodox faith:
- forbids the serving of milk and milk products with meats
- forbids cooking of food on the Sabbath
- forbids eating of leavened bread during Passover
- observes specific fast days

Daily Psychological Needs

- independence and security
- affection and love
- acceptance and social interaction
- trust and dignity
- self-esteem and relationships
- knowledge and achievement

FAMILY DYNAMICS

The family unit has changed over the past few decades. The primary family—mother, father, and children—is now frequently made up of step-parents, step-children, and half-brothers and sisters. The extended family—grandparents, aunts, and uncles—used to live in the same location, but are now scattered over large geographical areas. As travel became easier, families moved to separate parts of the country. Changes seen in the family unit have been the result of many factors such as:

- smaller families
- single-parent families
- divorces and second marriages
- interracial families
- two-career families
- same-sex households
- aging elderly
- baby boomers
- multicultural families
- diversity and blending of ethnic groups

Given all of these factors, the **family dynamics** in the home are also greatly influence. Other factors contributing to differences in the family that may affect the client include:

- increase in medical technology
- growth of new minority groups
- blend of cultures in diet, religion, and customs
- differences in health practices and beliefs
- family structure
- language and communication barriers

All of these factors and differences may influence the client and family's behavior. Acceptance by the health care members is the key to understanding these differences. However, if the HCA believes the behavior may in some way interfere with the client's recovery, it is important to report this to the supervisor.

family dynamics   the interaction among family members.

Helpful Hints: Sometimes taking a little time to get to know the client and his or her culture will prove to be a foundation for trust.

impairments disorders that affect normal function.

COMMUNICATION

Of all the factors affecting the relationships and interactions between client and family and the HCA, communication is so important it requires further discussion. The United States is a melting pot of many cultures with many different languages and various methods of communication. In addition, the client with diabetes may have visual **impairments** which can create even more problems in the communication process.

Proper communication is not only what is said but the way in which it is expressed, and includes gestures and facial expressions. A positive and cheerful attitude, which is also professional, promotes a trusting relationship between the HCA and the client (Figure 11–3).

Some general guidelines to improve communication skills are:

- Attitude should be calm and supportive.
- Touch, and caring behavior are effective reassurances.
- Eye contact should be maintained.
- Speaking should be slow and distinct, with a lower pitch and tone.
- Only one question should be asked at a time, and plenty of time allowed for responses.
- Communication should show respect and dignity to the client, especially the elderly and disabled.
- Speaking should be slow when conversing with friends and family; each word must be spoken clearly, especially when speaking to someone hard of hearing or to someone whose native language is not English.

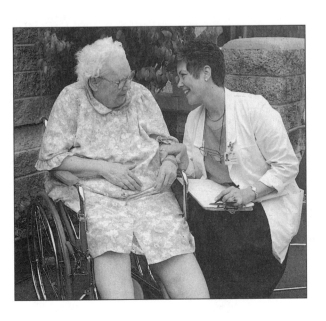

Figure 11–3 The HCA's body language shows the client she cares, and is interested in what the client has to say.

- HCAs should learn to listen. and be patient until the message is completed by the sender, even if the sender has a difficult time stating the message; time spent here is time saved later.

- When talking with persons from another culture, HCAs should not try using the words and phrases from different cultures as some of the words and phrases may have special meanings unless the client or family wishes to teach special vocabularies and words. In this case, setting up an agreed-upon mode of communication can be helpful.

- Reporting and recording of events should be done in simple terms and sentences.

Communicating with the elderly is vital in gaining information important to the nurse and/or physician. However, the HCA must remember that the elderly think and speak more slowly than other clients, and must not be rushed. Noise and distractions should be kept to a minimum, and short, simple words and sentences used. The nurse will determine if the client has impairments such as hearing, speech, or visual problems.

Hearing Impairments.

The hearing impaired present a special situation for the HCA. Table 11–2 identifies some common hearing changes and ways the HCA can help clients with these losses.

Supportive Communication Techniques

1. Speak clearly, slowly, in good lighting, and directly facing the hearing impaired client.

2. Be sure to get the client's attention before speaking. Do not start to speak abruptly.

3. Lower the pitch of your voice. Telephone bells, doorbells, horns, and emergency alarms should be at lowered tones.

Table 11–2 Hearing Changes and Ways to Help. (Courtesy: Glantz-Richman Rehabilitation Associates, Ltd.)	
Hearing Changes	**Ways to Help**
• There is a decline in auditor acuity with age called presbycusis. This age-related hearing loss is usually greater in men than in women. The reason for this decline is not known, but it is suspected that men are exposed to more damaging noise during their lifetimes, possibly resulting from being in the military service or due to the nature of their jobs.	• Any older person may need your help in compensating for hearing loss. While people with visual impairments can compensate by bringing things closer, those with hearing loss cannot similarly compensate. • Speak slowly and clearly, and do not change the topic abruptly. Be sure to face the person at eye level and have light on your face so lipreading is possible. Ask the person what you can do to make hearing easier.

continues

Table 11–2 (continued)	
Hearing Changes	**Ways to Help**
• Hearing loss is worse at high frequencies, meaning that some sounds are heard while others are not. Sounds may be distorted, or heard incorrectly, and thus misinterpreted.	• Try to lower you voice rather than allowing your voice to become high or shrill. Women should be especially careful about this. • A sound system used for music, entertainment, or oral presentations should be adjusted so that the bass and lower tones are predominant.
• People with normal hearing have a wide range between the quietest sound they hear and the loudest, which is painful or irritating. For people with hearing loss, this range may be much narrower. Sounds may have to be quite loud to be heard, and sensitivity is increased. If sounds are even a little louder, they may be too loud to be understood or may even be painful.	• Talk to those people with hearing impairments to find out the optimum tone to use. Do not assume that simply making things louder will solve the problem. • Be aware of the fact that noise or music may be irritating and may cause anxiety for persons with hearing loss, even if it has no effect on you. Be especially aware of this situation when you are working with people who are unable to communicate their needs to you. Note signs of anxiety, and try changing noise levels.
• Hearing loss is greater of consonants than for vowels. S, Z, T, F, and G sounds are particularly difficult to discriminate, which causes difficulty in hearing words correctly. Words that are similar can be particularly difficult to discriminate.	• People should be aware of the fact that even if sounds can be heard, they may not always be heard correctly. The suggestions previously mentioned can be followed; in addition, it is helpful to limit the competing stimuli of background noise. Choose a quiet, private place for talking.
• Some hearing deficits can be helped by the use of hearing aids, but these must be worn and adjusted correctly to help. They also regularly require new batteries. Some people never learn to use their hearing aids correctly, or they do not get new batteries often enough	• Older persons can purchase hearing aids from reputable firms and should learn their proper use. Family members or caregivers serving older persons also should learn how to help adjust or insert the aid or how to change batteries when it is necessary.
• Some hearing deficits cannot be helped by hearing aids, and the person's hearing is so poor that verbal communication is difficult.	• Encourage the use of nonverbal communication such as big smiles, waving, pointing, or demonstrating. Offer opportunities for activity and social interaction that require no spoken communication. for example, cooking and cleaning up can be done in complete silence by two or more people who have good understanding and cooperation. Also, use writing as a form of communication. Those who appear to be very impaired can understand written statements and questions.
• Hearing and following a conversation can take tremendous amounts of effort and energy for someone with hearing loss. Motivation, the context of the environment and general feelings of well-being and energy can make a difference in the ability to understand verbal communication. Lack of any or all of these may result in apparent "selective hearing."	• We should try to be more tolerant of "selective hearing." This syndrome is often annoying for those who interact with people with hearing loss, but in some cases there may be some legitimate reasons for it to occur. • Provide opportunities for people to participate in activities that are enjoyable but require little conversation—for example, playing card, doing puzzles, preparing food, and taking walks.

continues

Table 11–2 (continued)	
Hearing Changes	**Ways to Help**
• Depression and paranoid reactions are common among older persons with hearing loss. When they cannot hear what is being said, they may begin to think that people are talking about them and saying negative things.	• Do everything possible to compensate hearing loss and to ensure that people know what is going on and what the conversation is about. If the conversation does not concern them, tell them what the topic is so that they will not feel left out or talked about.
• Hearing is important to more than communication. It is a way of getting signals from the environment, so it also relates to safety.	• People who work or live with a person with hearing loss should keep this in mind. People in the community also should realize that when an older person crosses the street, he or she may not hear a car horn.

Helpful Hints: Persons who have difficulty hearing are very sensitive about their impairment. Be careful not to laugh or make fun of their mistakes.

4. Repeat what is said using different words, when necessary.

5. Know in which ear the client has better hearing, and try to speak to that side.

6. Recognize that hearing decline can be a normal aspect of aging. Convey this understanding through your supportive attitude.

7. Help family members or those who work with older clients become better speakers by pointing out helpful speech habits such as those listed here.

Nonsupportive Communication Techniques

1. Shouting only increases nonintelligible sounds. Increasing the loudness grossly distorts what the client hears.

2. Do not conduct conversations where background noise, such as traffic or many persons talking at once, can interfere with hearing.

3. Speaking too softly, running words together, or looking away from the listener while speaking to a hearing-impaired client.

4. Nonsupportive behaviors that interfere with lipreading include:

   • exaggerated and distorted speech movements by persons trying to help the lipreader.

   • speech that is too rapid

   • poor lighting on the speaker's face

   • mustaches that cover the lip

   • anything covering the speaker's mouth such as cigars, pencils, fingers, food, or gum

Visual Impairments

Working with clients who have visual impairments is another special situation that requires good communication techniques geared for that particular situation. Diabetic clients are more likely to have vision problems due to chronic complications associated with the disease. Table 11–3 shows some common visual impairments and ways the HCA can help.

Table 11–3 Vision Changes and Ways to Help. (Courtesy: Glantz-Richman Rehabilitation Associates, Ltd.)

Vision Changes	Ways to Help
• As a person ages, the lens in the eye yellows and thickens. The muscles that control pupil size also weaken. As a result, the older eye requires more light than the younger eye. To see clearly, a 65-year-old eye needs more than twice as much light as a 20-year-old eye.	• Provide adequate lighting. Be aware of poor lighting and that the older person may be unable to see obstacles, read signs, or recognize familiar people when the lighting is poor.
• The lens grows unevenly and becomes striated. The lens tends to refract the light that passes through it, causing glare problems. A small amount of glare that may hardly bother a younger person may cause great difficulties for the older person. Glare also may cause anxiety and inability to concentrate.	• Carefully adjust shades or drapes throughout the day to avoid glare from windows. Avoid shiny surfaces that reflect light. Tabletops, waxed floors, vinyl upholstery, and mirrors may create glare. • Sunglasses, big-brimmed hats, or sunshades may help when clients are outdoors or riding in a car. When clients cannot express themselves, caregivers must watch for signs of anxiety due to glare.
• Changes in the lens make color perception more difficult. Pastel colors (pink, yellow, pale blue) may all look alike. Brown, dark blue, and black may be difficult to identify correctly.	• Do not interpret inability to identify colors as a sign of confusion. • Do not expect older people to use pastels and very dark colors in a color-coding system. Clients should not depend upon color to help them take the correct pill.
• The older eye does not adapt quickly to changes in light levels. Abrupt changes can be hazardous and may cause falls and other accidents.	• Place lights strategically and keep some lights on so that changes in lighting will be more gradual. For example, nightlights in bedrooms will help. • When there is an abrupt change in the light level, an older person should wait until the eyes have adapted before continuing to walk. • Be careful when placing furniture just inside any entryway. An older person who enters a building may bump into things that are just inside the door if his or her eyes have not yet adjusted to the change in lighting.

continues

Table 11–3   (continued)

Vision Changes	Ways to Help
• Conditions of the eye that cause vision loss are very common among older people. However, most older people are not totally blind and can be taught to use their residual vision. More than half of the severe visual impairments occur in people 65 and over. Legal blindness is most common in this age group. The changes in vision occur slowly, and older people are often unaware of them.	• Older people should have their eyes examined by an ophthalmologist regularly. • Moving closer to things is one of the best ways to see them better. • Extra-large things are easier to see. These include large-print dials, controls, and buttons. • Contrasting colors make things easier to see. For example, doorways can contrast with the wall, wall sides can contrast with the tablecloth, the chair seat can contrast with the floor, and personal items can contrast with a covering on the dresser top. • Avoid clutter. It is difficult to distinguish crowded items. • Don't change the furniture arrangement unless it is necessary; if you do, ensure that older people become familiar with the new layout.
• Glaucoma is an insidious eye disease that has no noticeable symptoms until irreversible damage is done. It involves a loss of vision due to raised intraocular pressure, which damages the optic nerve. Glaucoma can be controlled and vision loss prevented if it is detected in time.	• There is currently a simple and painless test for glaucoma that older adults should be made aware of. They also should realize the importance of having the test.
• At this time there is no known prevention for cataracts, but they can be successfully treated by the surgical removal of the lens that has become cloudy and opaque. The surgery is usually performed when the vision loss has become severe. The lack of a natural lens in the eye is compensated for by special optical lenses that can be recognized by their thickness and the magnification of the person's eyes behind them.	• If a person has had cataract surgery and wears the special glasses, he or she may still experience some difficulty seeing. The person may need help reading, crossing the street, and doing other things that we assume should be easy. Those wearing the special lenses also may be unsure of themselves and want extra reassurance or assistance. However, people who are very proud may need extra assistance but may refuse to ask for it. Ask people how they might be assisted.
• Cataract glasses make objects seem larger. It is sometimes difficult for an older person to adjust to these distortions. A person wearing cataract glasses also has a blind spot at each side where the glasses cannot provide correction. This situation causes things to appear suddenly—to pop into a person's visual field. There is a new technique of implanting a lens in the eye at the time of surgery that has proven very successful. With implanted lenses, some of the problems of visual field change and size distortions are solved.	• Some people are self-conscious about the fact that the lenses make their eyes appear large and may need reassurance. • To avoid startling someone who wears cataract glasses, approach slowly from the front, rather than from the side.
• Macular degeneration is a condition that causes loss of central vision as the macula, the area of the retina responsible for central vision, deteriorates. This	• It may be reassuring to tell the person that he or she will not be totally blind from the disease but will retain peripheral vision.

continues

Table 11–3 (continued)

Vision changes	Ways to help
condition is neither preventable nor curable. It will not, however, cause total blindness because peripheral vision is not affected. A current method being tested to slow the advance of macular degeneration uses a laser to cauterize the hemorrhaging blood vessels in the retina.	• Low-vision aids such as magnifying glasses can be of some help to those in the less-advanced stages of macular degeneration. • Persons with macular degeneration may seem not to have a severe vision problem. Due to their peripheral vision, they can move around independently without bumping into things and may appear to see quite well. When they talk about their vision problems, other people may not believe them and think they are looking for unnecessary extra help or attention.
• There is some indication that a relationship exists between visual loss and mental function.	• Compensation and correction for vision problems may possibly lead to better mental functioning. It is worth a try.
• Persons who have visual deficits are unable to benefit from the nonverbal feedback important to communication. They cannot see the smiles, frown, or other facial expressions that are an important part of conversation.	• When conversing with persons who have vision problems, use touch to compensate. For example, holding, squeezing, or patting someone's hand lets the person know where you are and assures the person that you have not walked away.
• Dining can present special problems for people with visual impairments. These people may have difficulty eating independently or be afraid to dine socially because they might spill or make mistakes. Food that is difficult to see is not appealing.	• For those with low vision, place settings should be uncluttered, colors should contrast, and glare should be limited. A tablecloth or place mat can lessen glare. Someone should name the foods and tell where each is located. Finger foods and snack time should be provided regularly to allow people to feel more comfortable about their ability to eat appropriately.
• Those who have vision problems may be unsure of themselves in social situations and may even be fearful if they are in unfamiliar surroundings and situations.	• Help people with vision problems to look attractive, and reassure them honestly about their appearance. Always explain the layout of a room and describe the people who are present and those who will accompany them to social activities. Do not leave them alone until they have someone they can talk with or until they are touching a table, chair, or wall that will help with their orientation.

The following are some guidelines for the HCA to remember when caring for clients with visual impairments:

1. If the client has glasses, make sure they are clean, and that he or she wears them. Also, make sure that glasses are in good repair and fit correctly.

2. Provide adequate lighting at all times. Pools of bright light among darkened areas or variations in light intensity should be avoided.

3. Reduce glare by avoiding shiny surfaces, waxed floors, and exposed light bulbs. Have shades or sheer curtains at windows to reduce glare.

4. Brightly colored rims on dishes reduce spills.

5. Sharply contrasting colors for doors, bedspreads, floors, and walls help clients find their way and reduce accidents.

6. Large print newspapers, magazines, and books should be provided.

7. Refer to positions on the face of a clock to help the client locate items on a dinner plate or tray.

8. Clients with decreased peripheral vision may not see people or items sitting beside them.

9. Black telephones with white numerals are easier to see. Telephones with large numbers and letters on the dial are available.

10. Do not move personal belongings or furniture without the client's knowledge.

11. Use sensory stimulation of sound, touch, and smell.

12. Use large clocks, clocks that chime, and radios to keep the client oriented to time.

13. Obtain talking books and other low-vision aids.

14. Numerals on doors and dials (such as a stove) should be large enough for clients with eye impairments to see or feel.

15. Magnifying glasses can be used.

16. Give simple instructions and explanations for anything you plan to do such as moving the client.

17. Glare is worse on rainy days or when there is snow. Sunglasses, sunvisors, caps, or hats with brims may help.

Speaking Impairments (Aphasia)

Communicating with clients who have difficulty in speaking (aphasia) creates another health care challenge. Clients who have strokes are slow to regain their speaking abilities, and require increased patience on the part of the HCA. Some important principles to remember in this situation include:

1. When helping a client learning to speak, your rate of speaking should be reduced by prolonging the pauses between words and phrases.

2. The urge to speak louder may be great when clients do not seem to understand. Do not yell; instead, speak in your normal voice; emphasize the main ideas and use gestures to help clarify meanings.

3. It is better to ask questions that can be answered "yes" or "no" when requiring reliable information. If the HCA wants to know what the client had to drink for dinner, ask "Did you have milk?" instead of "Did you have milk, coffee, or tea?"

Helpful Hints: The HCA should be alert to vision problems when clients try to read medication labels. This can often lead to medication errors.

4. One of the easiest pitfalls is to try to anticipate the next word the client is going to use, and supply it. Do not supply the word unless the client requests it, since the aphasia may cause frustration or embarrassment.

5. Talking about a client in his or her presence is rude, and may also be discouraging. Aphasic clients especially, may understand, but be unable to express their thoughts and feelings.

6. It seems to be common nature for people to correct others' errors in speaking. Instead, be accepting of errors, understanding that speech and language will improve given time and proper training.

7. Never speak to adult clients as though they were children. Doing so creates hurt feelings that could lead to frustration and depression, or feelings of resentment against the speaker. Adult clients, regardless of their abilities, are not children and do not deserve to be treated as such.

8. Do not attempt to continue tasks that are frustrating to the client for long periods of time. Aphasic clients may have a reduced ability to attend to activities for long periods of time and tire quickly. Arrange for short periods of activity, and seek improvements in small steps so that some successes can be achieved.

9. Discourage clients from remaining alone all day. When possible, clients should have opportunities to interact with others, in order to see that they can be accepted and enjoy life, despite their aphasic difficulties.

10. Give positive reinforcement (both verbal and nonverbal) to the client's progress.

The ultimate goal in communicating with home care clients is to provide the best ongoing care possible. Sometimes this means making changes in care based on the information the HCA sees and hears. The information might help provide better care, or it could go through the supervisor and serve as a suggestion to change the care plan. If the changes are serious enough, perhaps the supervisor will speak to the doctor to reevaluate the orders.

STRESSES ON THE ELDERLY CLIENT

The following is a list of factors that can cause stress to the elderly client, and which may influence his or her recovery:

- disturbance in sleep
- loss of friends
- loneliness
- fear of illness
- loss of a beloved pet

- decreasing eyesight
- decreasing hearing
- fear of illness
- loss of metal abilities
- fear of impending death
- economic losses and concerns
- loss of driver's license
- fear of hospitalization
- illness of significant other
- feelings of dependency
- wish for more family visits
- less ability to care for oneself
- death of a family member or close friend
- use of assistive devices
- loss of prior social or recreational activities
- regrets
- missing children

BEHAVIORS OF THE HCA

confidentiality keeping all client information private.

Confidentiality means that information about the client and/or family is personal and should not be repeated to persons outside of the workplace. The HCA must follow the basic guidelines for confidentiality:

- discuss the client's medical and personal facts *only with the health care team*.
- *never* give out the client's medical information.
- do not discuss coworkers or workplace problems with peers or family; go to the supervisor.
- do not discuss personal activities in front of the client (Figure 11–4).

Helpful Hints: Clients in nursing homes or acute care living facilities are very curious about other clients and their private lives. Be courteous but definite about not giving personal information about one client to another.

HCA Attitudes

cultures the embodiment of ethnic backgrounds, including foods, beliefs, ethics, and lifestyles.

HCAs also come from many **cultures** and backgrounds, and each HCA brings his or her ethics and code of behavior to the home which is his or her workplace. These include:

- honesty with peers and clients
- respect of the home as a guest
- acceptance of differences in families
- reporting abuse
- caring of yourself and your appearance

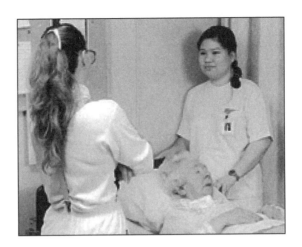

Figure 11–4 The HCA should not discuss personal activities in front of the client.

- knowing and respecting the client's rights
- keeping a cheerful and positive attitude
- being dependable and on time
- never leaving the workplace with work unfinished
- not accepting tips or gifts
- knowing the HCAs rights

  Positive attitudes that reflect HCAs of the highest level are:

- cheerful at tasks
- smiling during visits
- happy to do "extras"
- pride in appearance
- follows directions well
- empathetic to the client
- praises even small client participation
- leaves personal problems at home

All persons with disabilities should be given the opportunity to live at the highest level of self-care and self-respect, and in a safe and healthy environment.

REVIEW QUESTIONS

1. Four barriers to the relationship between the HCA and the client or family are:

    a.

    b.

    c.

    d.

2. Multicultural differences may occur in which area?
   a. race
   b. religion
   c. language
   d. all of the above

3. Examples of human physical needs are all but which of the following?
   a. food
   b. water
   c. love
   d. rest

4. Which is *not* a psychological need?
   a. safety
   b. affection
   c. trust
   d. dignity

5. Which of the following are examples of factors contributing to differences in families that may affect the client?
   a. language
   b. technology
   c. cultures
   d. baby boomers

6. True or False? The HCA's acceptance of differences is important for the client relationship.

7. True or False? The HCA may discuss medical information with the family.

8. True or False? Anger is a typical client response to a disability.

9. True or False? Decreasing numbers of friends is a source of stress for the elderly client.

10. True or False? The elderly do not feel stressed or concerned about increasing dependency on others.

11. True or False? Touch can be an effective means of communication.

12. True or False? If the client or family wish to teach the HCA some cultural phrases, they should refuse.

13. Unscramble the following key term from the chapter: mipienmatr _____

Glossary

abuse   the physical or psychological harm inflicted on one person by another; it may or may not be intentional

Acetest®   a simple urine test done to test for ketone bodies

acute   severe, but of short duration

advocate   a supporter; one who supports another person

aerobic exercises   exercises designed to increase the heart rate and provide increased oxygen and improved circulation to the body

aseptic   free of germs

carbohydrates   compounds of carbons, hydrogens, and oxygen, such as sugars and starches; most are formed by green plants

cardiovascular disease   any abnormal condition related to the heart and its blood vessels.

chronic complication   an illness or disorder that develops slowly over time, but may last for the client's lifetime

Clinitest®   a simple urine test for glucose levels; less accurate than blood glucose monitoring

complex carbohydrates   come from starch sources and are slow to be changed to blood glucose

complications   a second disease, or abnormal condition, occurring during the course of the primary disease

confidentiality   keeping all client information private

confused   disturbed orientation to time, place, and person

cultures   the embodiment of ethnic backgrounds, including foods, beliefs, ethics, and lifestyles

disoriented   a state of mental confusion as to time, place, and identity

documentation   the written account of what is seen, heard, and observed by the HCA

exploitation   a situation in whicn one person takes unfair advantage of another person

family dynamics   the interaction among family members

flammable   able to catch fire

gangrene   decay and death of tissue as a result of poor or no circulation to a body part

glands   groups of cells that produce secretions

glucagon   hormone that increases blood sugar and opposes the effects of insulin

glucose   natural sugar in foods

glucose self-monitoring   the client able to perform glucose testing on himself or herself by using an at-home device

HCA Care Plan   the plan written by the nurse-in-charge specifying the care to be provided by the HCA on each client visit

holistic caring model   a treatment method in which physical, emotional, psychological, ethical, and cultural considerations all play a role

hormones   substances formed in glands and carried to organs or tissues to carry out specific bodily functions

hyperglycemia   high blood sugar

hypoglycemia   low blood sugar

hypoglycemic coma   a condition caused by low levels of sugar in the bloodstream

impairments   disorders that affect normal function

incontinence   inability of a person to control bowel or bladder function

infection   illness resulting from the entrance into the body of a pathogen through ingestion, inhalation, or physical contact

insulin   hormone that helps the body utilize sugar and carbohydrates

insulin shock   shock as a result of excessive amounts of insulin in the blood

insulin therapy   control of a diabetic patient with the use of insulin

intervention   interceding on behalf of one person by another

islets of Langerhans   cells in the pancreas which produce the hormones insulin and glucagon

ketoacidosis   ketone bodies containing acetone spill into the bloodstream

limitations   restriction of activity

myocardial infarction (MI)   a heart attack

nephropathy   a disease affecting the kidneys

neuropathy   a disease affecting the nervous system

obesity   the state of being overweight

oral hypoglycemic agents (OHAs)   oral medications that boost the pancreas to produce insulinl

palpitations   excessive pounding of the heart

pathogens   microbes which cause infection

periheral vascular disease (PVD)   disease affecting the blood vessels

podiatrist   a doctor who specializes in foot care

retinopathy   a disese affecting the retina of the eye

safe environment   an environment free of hazards to prevent illness or injury

self-abuse   the injury or pain to which a person subjects himself or herself

simple carbohydrates   come from sugar sources and are quickly changed to blood glucose

Somogyi effect   the sudden rise in blood sugar levels early in the morning

Index

Page numbers followed by *f* or *t* denote figures or tables

A

Abuse of the elderly, 104–112
    defined, 106
    factors contributing to, 107–108
    prevention, 110–111
    reporting, 107
    signs of
        behavioral signs, 108–109
        environmental signs, 109
        physical signs, 108
    substance abuse, 110
    types of
        active neglect, 107
        material/financial, 107
        passive neglect, 106
        physical, 107
        psychological, 106
        self-abuse/self-neglect, 107
Acetest®, 70
Acetone, testing for, with KetostixR, 70–71
Active neglect, 107
Acute, defined, 40
Adrenal glands, 2f
    function of, 3
Advocate, 114
Aerobic exercises, 83
Airborne transmission, 101
Air mattress, 61
Alcohol consumption, 81
American Diabetes Association (ADA), diet, principles and restrictions
    of, 75–76, 79–80
Amputations, 48
Antidiuretic hormone, 11
Aphasia, 124–125
Aseptic practices, 102–103
Assistive devices to prevent pressure sores, 61
Attitudes of the HCA, 126–127

B

Baths and showers, 62
Bed cradle, 61
Behaviors of the HCA, 126
Biotin, 78t
Bladder training, 63–65
    procedure, 65, 68
    retraining assessment, 66–67f
Blindness, 12t, 122t
Body fat, calculating, 80
Body substance isolation, 101
Bowel training, 63–65
    enemas, 63
    procedure, 63–64
        suppositories, 63

C

Calorie, 75t
Carbohydrates, 20
    complex vs. simple carbohydrates, 81
    definition/examples of, 75t
    level of, when to change, 82t
    rapid-acting, for hypoglycemic reaction, 78
Cardiovascular disease, 48
    defined, 48
    prevention guidelines for, 49
Cardiovascular system, 5, 6f
Care plan, 32, 33f, 34, 35f
Cataracts, 49, 122t
Causes of diabetes, 14
Cerebrovascular accidents (CVA), 4
Children, diabetes in, 11–12
Client care procedures, 54–72
    bladder training, 65–68
    bowel training, 63–65
    collecting a fresh, fractional urine specimen, 68–69
    foot and toenail care, 56–58
    skin care and pressure sores, 58–63
    testing urine and blood sugar levels, 69–71
Clinitest®, 69–70
Cobalamin, 78t
Coma
    hyperglycemic, 43–44, 45t
        vs. insulin shock (hypoglycemic coma), 44, 45t
    ketoacidotic, 42
Communication, 117–126
    hearing impairments, 118–120
    improving communication skills, 117–118
    speaking impairments (aphasia), 124–125
    visual impairments, 121–124
Complications, ix, 6f, 12t, 12–13, 38–46
    acute
        hyperglycemia, 42–44
        hypoglycemia, 40
        insulin shock, 44–45
        ketoacidosis, 41–42
    chronic, 46–53
        cardiovascular disease, 48–49
        defined, 48
        eye disorders, 49, 121–124
        foot complications, 50
        gum disease, 51
        infections, 49–50
        neuropathy, 49
        prevention guidelines for, 52
        skin breakdown, 50–51
        stress, 51–52
    defined, 12
    education of the client about, 82

Confidentiality, 126
Confused, 96
Constipation
    See also Bowel training
    causes of, 64
    prevention of, 63

D

"Dawn phenomenon," 79
Depends™, 60
Depression, hearing loss and, 120*t*
Diabetes
    in children, 11–12
    classification of
        Diabetes Insidious Type V, 11
        Diabetes Insipidus Type IV, 11
        Gestational Diabetes Type III, 11
        Insulin-dependent (IDDM) Type I, 10
        Non-insulin-dependent (NIDDM) Type II, 10–11
Diabetic diet
    ADA diet, principles and restrictions of, 75–76, 79–80
    alcohol consumption and, 81
    body fat, calculating, 80
    complex vs. simple carbohydrates, 81
    education of the client about, 74–82
    example of, 80
    food
        groups, 76
        label, 79*f*
        purchasing of, 81
        pyramid, 80*f*
    meals
        preparation of, 81
        skipping, 78
        timing of, guidelines for, 78
    nutritional terms, 75*t*
    rapid-acting carbohydrates, for hypoglycemic reaction, 78
    Somogyi effect, 79
    vitamins and sources of, 77–78*t*
Diagnosis of diabetes, 14–15
Diagnostic Related Groups (DRGs), ix
Dialysis, 5, 43
Diet. *See* Diabetic diet
Diseases requiring transmission-based precautions, 102*t*
Disoriented, 96
DKA. *See* Ketoacidosis, diabetic (DKA)
Documentation, 28, 36
    guidelines for, 31–32
Droplet transmission, 101
Drug-resistant organisms, 101

E

Education of the client
    about complications, 82
        carbohydrate level, when to change, 82*t*
    about diet, 74–82
    about exercise, 83–84
    social support, 84–85
Egg crate mattress, 61
Elbow pads, 60*f*
Endocrine system, 2–3
    structures of, 2*f*, 3
Enemas, 63
Equal™, 81
Exercise, 83–84
Exploitation, 107
Eye disorders, 4, 49
    See also Visual impairments

F

Falls, preventing, 91–93
Family dynamics, 116

Fasting blood sugar (FBS) test, 14, 20
Fats, definition/examples of, 75*t*
Fat-soluble vitamins, 77*t*
Finger-sticking device, 24*f*
Fire emergency measures, 96–98
    the fire extinguisher, using, 98
    first aid procedures for, 94*f*
    RACE system, 98, 99*f*
First aid procedures, for fire, 94*f*
Flammable, 91
Folacin, 78*t*
Food
    groups, 76
    label, 79*f*
    preparation of, 81
    purchasing of, 81
    pyramid, 80*f*
    sugar-free, 79
Foot and toenail care, 56
    complications, 50
    procedure, 56–58
Foot pads, 60*f*, 61*f*
Fungal infections, of the feet, 50

G

Gangrene, 12*t*
    defined, 50
Gel foam cushions, 61
Gestational Diabetes Type III, 11
Glands, 2
Glaucoma, 49, 122*t*
Glucagon, defined, 2
Glucose
    defined, 10
    effects of, 13
    management and control of, 16–25
        glucose self-monitoring, 23, 24*f*, 84
        insulin therapy, 18–21
        oral hypoglycemic agents, 21–22
    metabolism of, 20–21
    in urine, 5
        testing for, with Clinitest®, 69–70
Glucose self-monitoring, 23, 24*f*
    before and after exercising, 84
Glucose tolerance test, oral (OGTT), 14
Glycosylated hemoglobin AIC, 14
Gum disease, 51

H

HCA care plan, 32, 33*f*, 34, 35*f*
HCA roles and functions, 26–37
    attitudes of the HCA, 126
    behaviors of the HCA, 126
    care team, 34, 36*f*
    documentation, 31–32, 36
    new roles for the HCA, 34, 36
    observation and reporting, 28–30
    physical observation, 29
    telephone reporting, 30
    twelve areas of concern, 29–30
Hearing impairments, 118–120
    hearing changes and ways to help, 118–120*t*
    nonsupportive communication techniques, 120
    supportive communication techniques, 118, 120
Hemorrhoids, 64
Holistic caring model, 114–116
Hormones, 2, 20
Hyperglycemia, 10
    coma, 43–44
        vs. insulin shock, 44, 45*t*
    emergency measures for, 43
    signs and symptoms of, 21, 42–43
    Somogyi effect, 79
Hypertension, 5, 48
    exercising and, 84

Hypoglycemia, 20
    foods for episodes of, 40
    hypoglycemic shock (insulin shock), 41*f*
    vs. ketoacidosis, 41*f*
    rapid-acting carbohydrates for, 78
    signs and symptoms of, 40

I

IDDM. *See* Insulin-dependent (IDDM) Type I Diabetes
Identification tag, 15
Impaction, 64
Impairments, 117
Incontinence, 59, 63
Infection control, 98–103
    aseptic practices, 102–103
    diseases requiring transmission-based precautions, 102*t*
    medical terms about, 101–102
    personal protective equipment (PPE), 100–101
    standard precautions, 100, 101*f*
    universal precautions, 99
Infections, 49–50
Insulin-dependent (IDDM) Type I Diabetes, 10
Insulin shock (hypoglycemic shock)
    causes of, 44
    vs. diabetic coma, 44, 45*t*
Insulin therapy, 18–21
    See also Oral hypoglycemic agents (OHAs)
    actions of insulin, 4*f*, 20
    combination therapy, 22
    eye drops, 24
    illness and, 82
    injections, 18–19
        body areas for, 19*f*
    insulin defined, 2
    insulin pumps, 19, 24
    nasal spray, 24
    types of insulin, 19*t*
Intervention, 110
Islets of Langerhans, 2
    function of, 3
Itching, 13

J

Juvenile diabetes. *See* Insulin-dependent (IDDM) Type I Diabetes

K

Ketoacidosis, diabetic (DKA), 13
    vs. hypoglycemia, 41*f*
    ketoacidotic coma, 42
    signs and symptoms of, 41–42
Ketone bodies, urine testing for, with AcetestR, 70
Ketonuria, 41
KetostixR strip test, 70–71
Kidney disease, 5, 12*t*

L

Laboratory tests, 14, 70
    See also specific tests
Legs, diabetic effects to, 4
Limitations, 32

M

Macular degeneration, 122–123*t*
Material/financial abuse, 107
Meals
    preparation of, 81
    skipping, 78
    timing of, guidelines for, 78
Medic AlertR tag, 15*f*
Medical social worker (MSW), 84
Medication safety, 93
Metabolism, 75*t*
Minerals, definition/examples of, 75*t*
Multicultural differences, 116

Myocardial infarction (MI), 5
    defined, 13

N

Nephropathy, 12
    exercising and, 84
Nerve degeneration, 12*t*
Nervous system, 3–4, 5*f*
Neuropathy, 4
    defined, 12
    signs and symptoms of, 49
Niacin, 77*t*
Non-insulin-dependent (NIDDM) Type II Diabetes, 10–11

O

Obesity, 10
Oral glucose tolerance test (OGTT), 14
Oral hygiene, 51
Oral hypoglycemic agents (OHAs), 21–22
    problems associated with, 22
Ovaries, 2*f*
    function of, 3

P

Palpitations, 28
Pantothenic acid, 78*t*
Parathyroid glands, 2*f*
    function of, 3
Passive neglect, 106
Pathogens, 99
Peripheral vascular disease (PVD), 5
    complications of, 48
    defined, 12
Personal protective equipment (PPE), 100–101
Physical abuse, 107
Physical needs, 115
Physical observations, 29
Pituitary gland, 2*f*
    function of, 3
Podiatrist, 56
Polydipsia, 13
Polyphagia, 13
Polyuria, 13
Postprandial glucose test, two-hour, 14
Presbycusis, 118*t*
Pressure ulcers. *See* Skin care and pressure sores
Prevalence of diabetes, ix, 10
Procedures. *See* Client care procedures
Programmable, implantable medication systems (PIMs), 19, 24
Proteins, definition/examples of, 75*t*
Psychological abuse, 106
Psychological concerns, 51–52
Psychosocial influences, 112–128
    behaviors/attitudes of the HCA, 126–127
    communication, 117–126
    daily physical needs, 115
    daily psychological needs, 116
    family dynamics, 116
    the holistic caring model, 114–116
    religious dietary practices, 115*t*
    religious/spiritual needs, 115
    stresses on the elderly, 125–126
Pumps, insulin, 19, 24
Pyridoxine, 77*t*

R

RACE system in a fire emergency, 98, 99*f*
Religious dietary practices, 115*t*
Religious/spiritual needs, 115
Reservoir, 101
Retaliation, 107
Retinitis, 49
Retinopathy, 4, 49
    defined, 12

exercising and, 84
Riboflavin, 77t
Roles and functions of the HCA. *See* HCA roles and functions

S

Safe environment, 88–89, 90–93
Safety and emergencies, 86–104
    in the bathroom, 89, 92f
    emergency measures
        for fire, 96–98
            first aid procedures for, 94f
        plans for, 95–96
    emergency phone numbers, 89f
    falls, 91–93
    infection control, 98–103
    in the kitchen, 89–90
    maintaining a safe environment, 88–89, 90–93
    medication safety, 93
    most common hazards, 90–91
    potential risks, 88
Self-abuse/self-neglect, 107
Self-monitoring of glucose, 23, 24f
Sharps, disposal of, 71
Sheepskin wool pads, 61
Signs and symptoms of diabetes, 13
Skin breakdown, 50–51
    prevention of, 59–60
    stages of, 59
Skin care and pressure sores, 58–63
    assistive devices to prevent pressure sores, 61
    blisters/scratches/sores, 62
    elbow pads, 60f
    foot pads, 60f, 61f
    procedure, 61–63
    sites for pressure sores, 60
    skin breakdown, 50–51, 59–60
Skin lesions, 13
Snacks, 79
Social support for the diabetic, 84–85
Somogyi effect, 79
Speaking impairments (aphasia), 124–125
Standard precautions, 100, 101f
Stress, 51–52
    on the elderly client, 125–126
    management techniques for, 52
Stroke, 4
Substance abuse, in the elderly, 110
"Sugar-free" foods, 79

Sulfonylureas. *See* Oral hypoglycemic agents (OHAs)
Suppositories, 63
Surgery, risk of glucose imbalance and, 52
Sweeteners, alternative, 81
SweetOneTM, 81

T

Testes, 2f
    function of, 3
Thiamine, 77t
Thymus gland, 2f
    function of, 3
Thyroid gland, 2f
    function of, 3
Toenail care, procedure, 56–58
Total parenteral nutrition (TPN), 43
Transmission-based precautions, 101t

U

Ulcers, lower extremity, 48
Universal precautions, 99
Urinalysis, 14
Urinary system, 5, 6f
Urine testing
    for acetone, with Ketostix®, 70–71
    for glucose, with Clinitest®, 69–70
    for ketone bodies, with Acetest®, 70
    procedure, 68–69

V

Vaginitis, 13
Vascular disease, 12t
VaselineR, 56
Visit form, 35f
Visual impairments, 121–124
    guidelines for care, 123–124
    vision changes and ways to help, 121–123t
Vitamins
    definition/examples of, 75t
    sources and functions of, 77–78t

W

Water, definition of, 75t
Water mattress, 61
Water-soluble vitamins, 77–78t
Water temperature, for baths and showers, 62
Weakness, 13
Weight loss, 13